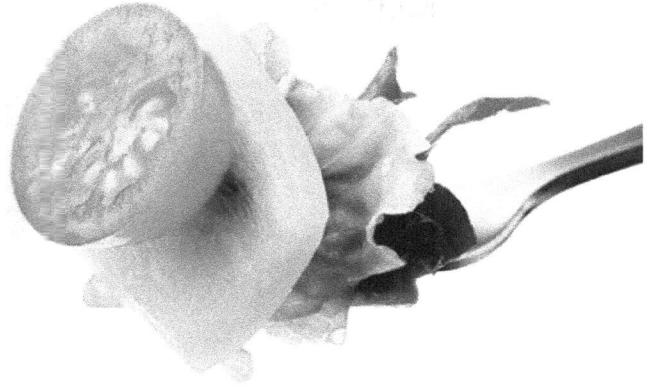

Medicine of Nature

Book of Recipies

Recipies that read like doctors prescriptions

Medicine of Nature 2. part

Mathias Mark Sanderson

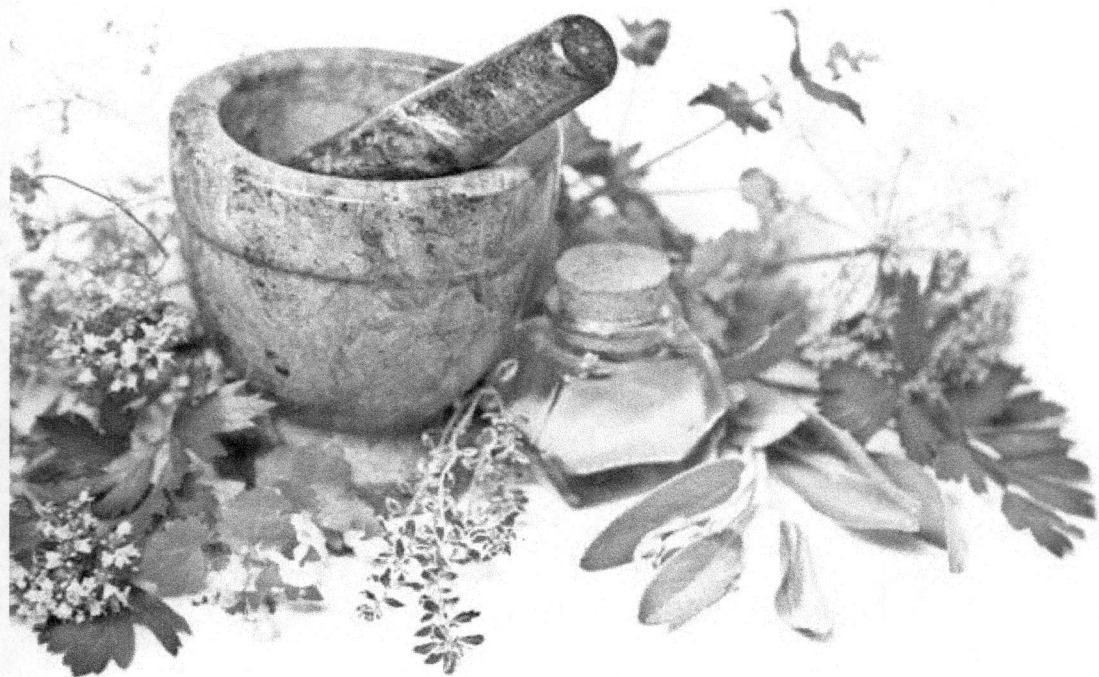

This is the first cookbook that combines raw and cooked food. It combines two different worlds; healthy raw food and classic cooking cuisine. On the one hand we have numerous cookbooks, which merely satisfy the taste, where health is not an issue, when we go through the numerous recipes for baking, frying and other ways of destroying vitamins and enzymes. On the other hand, there are those extreme 100% raw - fresh cookbooks intended only for a minority of enthusiasts. **This book is a bridge between the two worlds.** The recipes in it are intended for all, regardless of their nutritional beliefs or values. **Fresh food eaters will love the brilliant combinations, vegetarians will leap from joy because of the new discoveries and all-eaters will open their eyes in excitement. There is something for everyone, including the vegans.**

A WHOLE DIFFERENT STORY

A lot of cookbooks in the title promise "healthy cooking", but those promises soon fade when you read about sautéing the vegetables on olive oil or about a pie with withered baked blueberries. And as we flip through the pages, it becomes clear that there is no sign of healthy food. The criteria for healthy cooking are as clear as day. The preparation has to maintain all the vitamins, enzymes and minerals 100% intact or match this ideal as much as possible. Although laboratory tests show the chemical composition of vitamins, they don't show their properties which sustain life. Only raw food is rich in vitamins. Cooking marmalade and compotes is a mortal sin.

Healthy cuisine does not cook the fruit or bake it in pies or pastries; it doesn't destroy a single piece of fruit. It knows only natural sweeteners: honey, dates, raisins, agave nectar, but no sugar. Healthy cuisine uses 100% cold pressed oils, which are added at the end, nothing is frying in this oils. Healthy cuisine loves sweet and sour cream, cottage cheese, it worships different varieties of cheeses, but all strictly made from fresh milk, otherwise it is flirting with veganism. It hates pasteurization and does not use white flour. It likes whole-wheat flour, but mostly uses Kamut flour or khorasan wheat flour, or even prefers to sprout various grains. This is a completely different story, but the best is yet to come; the main part, the heart of this very special cookbook is explained in the following paragraph.

THE REVOLUTIONARY DIFFERENCE

In cooking it is common practice that all the ingredients go into one pot. Our recipes contain a revolutionary twist. The basic principle behind healthy cooking practice is to cook and bake only those ingredients, which are not edible raw, such as: potatoes, rice, peas, eggplants... All food which we can consume **raw, we shouldn't destroy with heat under any circumstances. Cooking tomatoes, spinach and carrots is a mortal sin.** We have to cook the rice and peas, but why also destroy the tomatoes, carrots, parsley and onions in the same pot? Cook the peas and rice separately, wait for it to cool off a bit and combine with finely chopped and pureed fresh vegetables – in this way we get a healthy risotto. This is the basic principle in all our recipes. **Healthy classic cuisine opens our eyes,** we do not have to give up culinary pleasures, we simply have to change the process, the technique of preparation. In this way classical culinary art and healthy food go hand in hand.

DON'T SWIM, IF THERE IS A BRIDGE IN FRONT OF YOU

All over the world there is a number of "dietetic nomads", who migrate from one diet to another. The research spirit is useful if one day we discover what works best and the right lifestyle for us. In the first part of the **Medicine of Nature - Global health reform,** I recommend minimum 75% raw diet, although I know from my personal experience that this is not easy. There are only a few people who actually live the raw food lifestyle, whereas most understand that this would be best, but habits and the environment draw them back to the other side. On the other hand, the state of affairs is not peachy. Statistically speaking, 90% of raw food eaters are somewhere between the two worlds and they are the ones who can mostly benefit from the bridge and cross over the temptation. In the future, a larger group of people will march down the highway of healthy food once the bridge is built.

FOR THE ENTIRE FAMILY

Healthy food nowhere else comes this close to the everyday life as it does in this book. **Most people don't want to eat only fresh - raw food, but still want a full plate of health. Contradictory, but true.** They wish to remain healthy, but don't want to give up the good food, popular dishes and social gatherings. **What now?** Then there are many individuals, who actually do eat healthy, but the rest of the family members don't wish to or are not interested in healthy food. With the recipes in this book, problem is solved. Without imposing they can show their families that healthy food can taste better than the food they are used to. Let them give it a taste and see for themselves. They will quickly demand more and acquire new habits for life. Good recipes can even smooth away the disagreements between family members, which are on different diets. Good recipes can connect people together.

COMBINED CULINARY AND MEDICAL RECIPES

If you read carefully, you will soon discover you are not merely reading culinary recipes for the preparation of food. On a piece of paper similar to the one you get at a doctor's visit, there are vitamins, minerals and enzymes prescribed, which can save your lives by correct and appropriate preparation. This happens when we combine the two sciences. A good doctor is a good dietician and an even better cook.

MOST USEFUL CHART

Charts with calories and nutritional values measured in grams per hundred grams for a nutrient barely have any practical value. You will not find these charts in this book, because they make no sense. The most useful chart is the one, which shows the food that can be consumed fresh and the food which is suitable for cooking. Below is the basic division, which you can complete over time, while preparing the recipes. Do not count the calories or over calculate because your body and the intelligence have other plans. The Chinese say 'Man-man-chi' ('Eat slow!') instead of 'Enjoy your meal'.

For cooking	Fresh - Raw
Potatoes	All fruit
Legumes	All dairy
Eggplants	products
Mushrooms	All fats
Peas	Tomato
Old corn	Spinach
Seldom onion	Carrot, parsley
Sometimes	Cauliflower
pumpkin	Broccoli
Exceptionally	Onion and Leek
fats	Parsley
	Artichokes
	Baby peas
	Baby corn
	Young zucchini

NEW GLOBAL STANDARDS

This book will cook up a storm. It will inspire many professional cooks, thousands of housewives all over the world and all who enjoy preparing food. Many food technologists will think again and change their minds. It sets new global standards for food processing. It carries the origins for a better tomorrow, for a new world. Before us is a rather different cookbook than we are used to. No doubt it is revolutionary, it will change our lives for all of us forever.

LET US TURN A NEW PAGE

How about a delicious marmalade without cooking?

How about 100% healthy puddings and ice-creams?

How would you like to toast with natural Schweppes?

How about enjoying pasta and pizza without feeling guilty?

Get your ladle, fork and spoon ready and let us cook up a storm...

RECEPIES

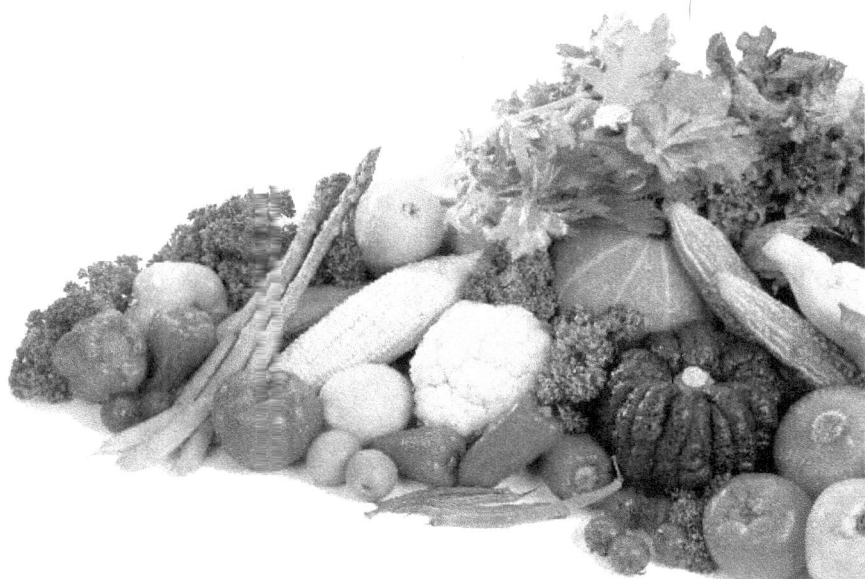

*Two cups of
natural C tea:
A fist of whole
rose hip (30-40g),
1 dl of rather warm water,
1 lemon,
1 orange,
2 ts of honey,
spices as desired:
vanilla,
cinnamon,
cardamom*

NATURAL C-TEA

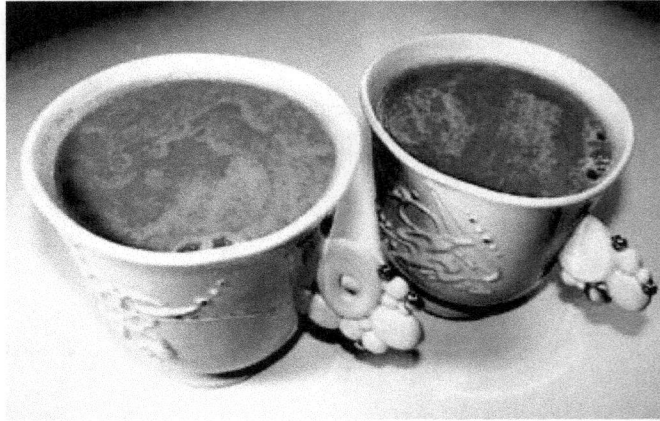

Albert Einstein once said that only two things are infinite: the universe and human stupidity. People do stupid things. Vitamin C is instantly destroyed in hot tea and on top of that at least a dozen other healing ingredients are destroyed in the process of cooking rose hip tea. When hot water becomes red coloured water, one takes the tea bag out and throws the best part away. When having a headache, one drives to the pharmacy to get Aspirin past rosehip bushes, which contain beautiful, miraculous red fruit. The tale of the sailors and scurvy is not over yet... Einstein's hairs on the back of his neck stand on ends.

Rose hip is the best natural Aspirin, surpassing all the pills on the market. A headache wears off within 5-10 minutes after drinking a cup of rose

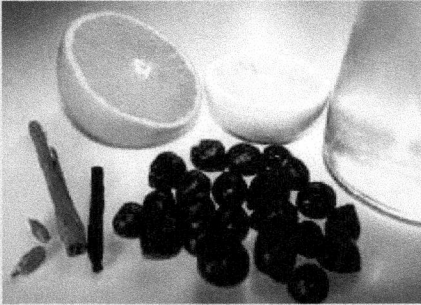

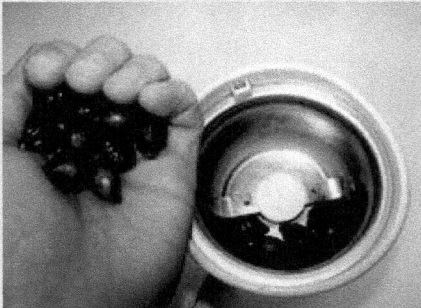

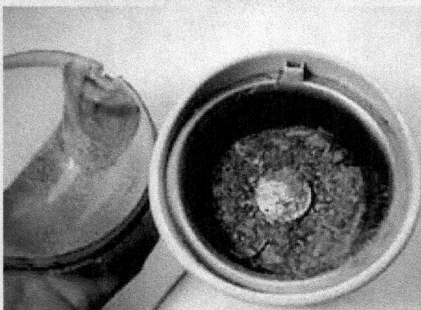

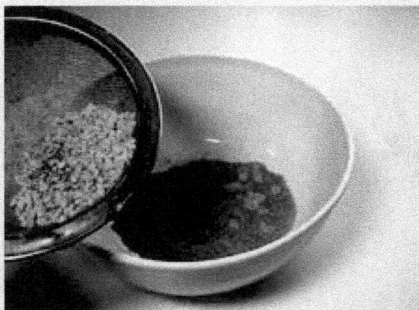

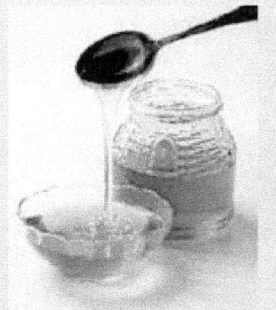

hip tea made according to this recipe. It is even more efficient, if we spend half an hour walking in the woods to get the oxygen we need before drinking the tea. Oxygen, vitamins and enzymes – this is what the body cells need! Rose hip, if prepared correctly, increases concentration as much as coffee, therefore it can easily replace it in the morning ritual. This type of coffee wakes us up, opens the breath, strengthens the senses and the heart beats in its natural rhythm, contrary to black coffee, which disturbs the heartbeat.

Let's learn how to make rose hip tea correctly: grind the rose hip in a coffee grinder real quick to get red powder mixed with whole seeds (app. 15 seconds). On a fine strainer sift it to lose the seeds and get only the healing powder. Put it back in the coffee mill and completely grind it (45 seconds). Sift it through a strainer and the magical powder is ready to make the tea. Squeeze an orange and lemon or other citruses, like mandarins. Mix the powder with the juice, honey and warm water, but beware - not hot! The tea should be at body temperature, we must not let the medicine be destroyed by the heat. In a couple of minutes we have made a super drink. With regular use you can rename the coffee grinder into a tea grinder. Even better if you have a flour grinder and grind the rose hip into fine powder. Pick the rose hip in late autumn, dry it at room temperature and conserve in glass jars, make a stock for the winter.

I discovered this healing rose hip tea by accident. One day, I simply couldn't wait for the rose hip to soak in hot water and for the tea to cool, so I took the coffee grinder, ground the rose hip and mixed it with warm water. The tea woke me up in an instant, as though I just woke up from a dream. I think I mumbled something, but can't remember what it was. It hit me, when I saw Einstein riding on a ray of light. He waved and said: "It's all relative, depends on how quickly you make the tea." The tea was made instantly and that's why it hit me. With a cup of this tea you can feel the real internal energy. It should be called Instant C tea or Einstein C tea, as the life expectancy of a person drastically prolongs with it.

The flavour of natural C tea is fantastic. It is a drink, which revivifys, a true vitamin drink, aspirin and the first drink, which you will get regardless of the condition in the hospitals of the future, as it greatly strengthens the immune system. Natural C tea in the form of fine powder packed in bags of 2-3g like sugar is soon going to be available in every supermarket anywhere and anytime. You will have it with you in your handbag instead of aspirin. There comes a time of great changes, when the mistakes of our ancestors will no longer be repeated. The change has already begun, turn to the next page.

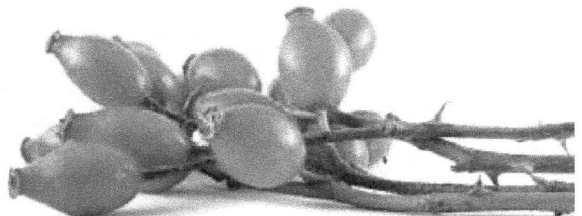

Plum jam:
250g prunes,
2dl water,
1-2 tbs honey,
if desired agar-agar

Strawberry jam:
250g dry strawberries,
2dl pure water,
2-4 ts of agave nectar

Mango jam:
200g dry mango,
4-5 jumbo dates,
2dl water, vanilla

Kamut pancakes:
250g Kamut flour,
1.5 dl of sparkling water,
4 dl of warm water,
salt,
ome coconut oil for baking fat

PANCAKES WITH PLUM, STRAWBERRY AND MANGO MARMALADE

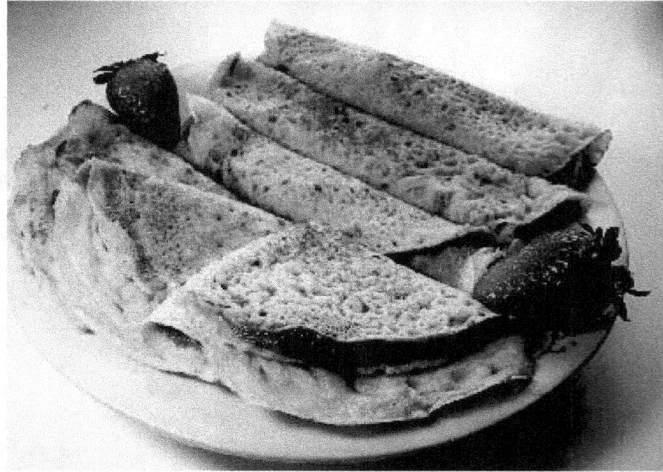

In conventional cuisine, the fruit is cooked for long hours, then white sugar is added and in this way a lot of diseases are cooked up. The taste is shallow, the flavours lost in the taste of sugar. Thickening of the fruit by cooking enhances the aroma, but destroys everything good in fruit. Marmalade without cooking? Yes, we can preserve 100% vitamins and 100% of living elements. Dry fruit marmalade is healthy, fully aromatic and much more tasteful.

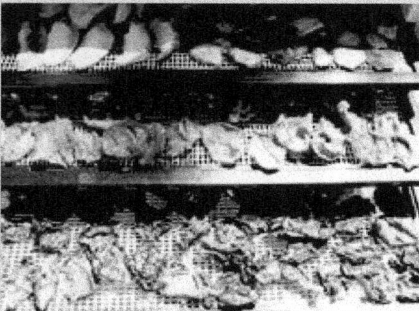

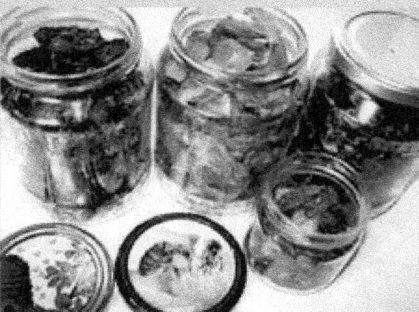

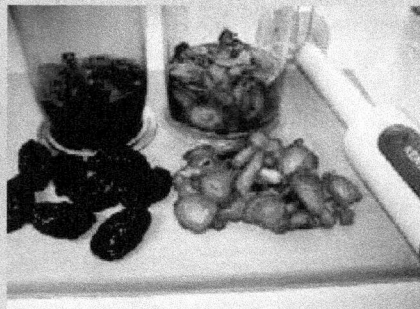

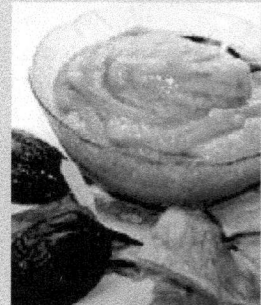

Preparation of natural marmalade is as simple as adding 1 + 1. Soak any dry fruit for 15-30 minutes in water, blend it with a blender and sweeten it with honey, agave nectar or mix in the dates. If you want real jam, mix it for a shorter period of time and stir several times, so to leave pieces of fruit. For jelly lovers boil an even spoon of agar in ½ dl of water, cool for thirty seconds and stir in with the marmalade than put it in fridge.

When I made plum marmalade in this way for the first time, I couldn't believe it. It was the best tasting marmalade I had ever had. I prepared strawberry, apricot, peach, blueberry and mango marmalade in the same way and.. loved it! Each was better than the previous one. These are heavenly marmalades! One particularly good is made from apricots and peaches. For blueberry marmalade the ratio is prunes : dry blueberries 50 : 50. You can use even fresh berries; any berries you can mix with dry dates, pruns, honey mixture. Try fresh strawberries with pruns and honey, or fresh mango and madjool dates.You can make rose hip marmalade if you soak a little rose hip powder and mix it with honey. Strawberry marmalade is best sweetened with agave nectar and mango with dates. Try your own mixtures, add a pinch of vanilla, experiment, get crazy, get wild...

You will have to dry the fruit yourself, because that, which is bought, except for certain exceptions and tropical fruit, is not useful, as it is dried at excessive temperatures and more or less cooked. Stone the fruit, slice into 6-7 mm slices and dry in a fruit drier at 42ºC. Drying has to be slow; it should last for 24 – 48 hours,

to preserve life. The fruit which contains lots of juice can initially be dried at higher temperatures (around 50ºC for 2-3 hours), then lower the temperature, because the water when it evaporates, cools the surface from where it evaporates, thus producing a cooling effect. We can speed up the drying in the beginning without destroying the life in the food. At the peak of the season stock up on dry fruit and then you can make fresh marmalade whenever you wish to, every day, once a week, a month... When the fruit is in season, do not hesitate to dry it, not necessarily in huge amounts; a couple of cases will be sufficient. Dry the fruit well before putting it in glass jars, which are to be kept in a cold place. Preparing for the winter will be different from now on.

The recipe for pancakes is also unique. Make the batter out of whole-wheat Khorasan Kamut flour, warm water, some sparkling mineral water and a pinch of salt. Khorasan or Kamut is a special sort of grain, better than wheat; therefore we don't need either eggs or milk. We wouldn't be alive, if we didn't break the rules just a bit, and in order to make pancakes we need a bit of fat. We have chosen coconut fat, which is stable at higher temperatures and adds flavour to the pancakes. You will love it, your grandma will love the new recipe and the entire family will be healthier.

The next time you decide to bake croissants, first of all, make them out of Khorasan wheat and second, make them empty, without marmalade. Bakers, listen up! Hotel chefs, especially those in five-star and deluxe hotels, serve your guests a healthy breakfast.

Spinach sauce:
500 g spinach,
2 dl unpasteurized sour cream
(for vegans half of avocado),
garlic clove,
5-6 tbs cold pressed sunflower oil,
salt

spices:
nettle,
parsley leaves with root,
rocket,
celery

Gnocchi:
750 g potatoes,
250 g Kamut flour,
salt

GNOCCHI WITH SPINACH SAUCE

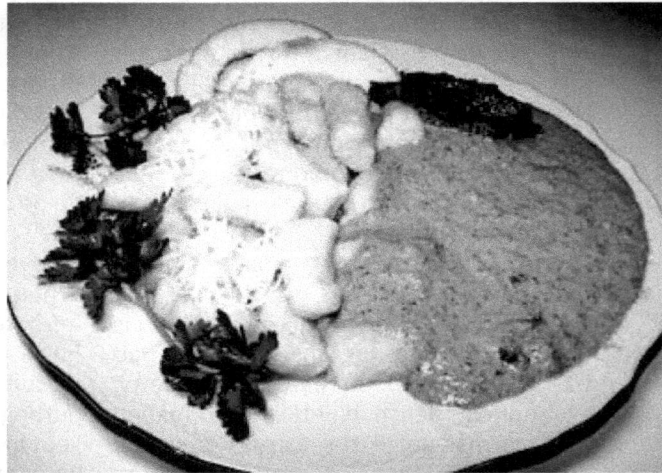

The Sun is the main chef on the planet Earth. When it shines its rays on the green spinach leaves, the inorganic elements become living organic substances in the leaves – the miracle of life occurs. If you cook the spinach, the living molecules become inorganic and life magically disappears. Spinach is very healthy, full of calcium, iron, folic acid, enzymes, but if you cook it, it becomes poison. In the process of cooking, the oxalic acid turns into calcium depriver. Instead of calcium building in the body, it is disappearing. Never, never cook spinach! Blanching is just as destructive.

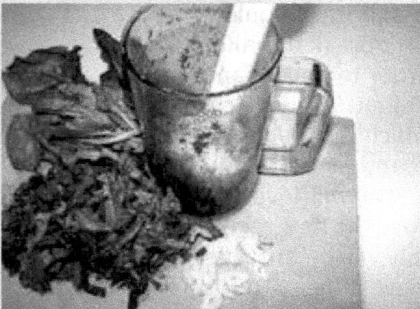

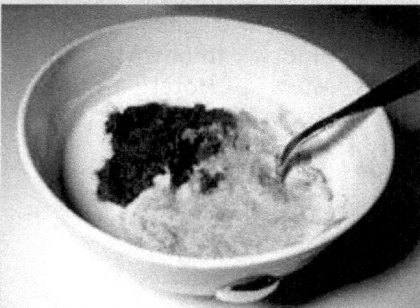

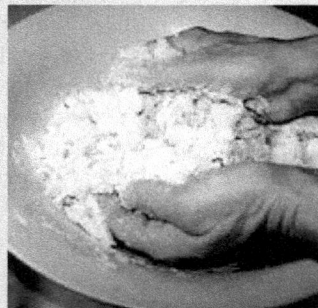

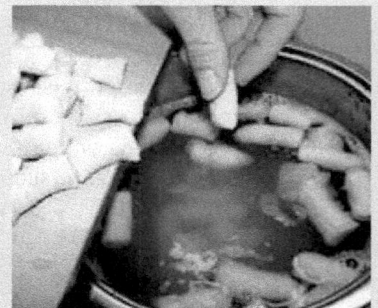

We can prepare the spinach without cooking, it is faster, tastes better and the minerals and vitamins remain intact and life continues to flow...

"Spinach sauce without cooking?" Really simple, as all great things usually are. Rinse the spinach, chop on a cutting board and blend into a puree. In the blender you cannot liquefy the spinach leaves without adding liquid, much less in a food processor, so use a powerful hand blender. Add a few spoons of oil to mix easily. You can mix some branches of nettle from the garden, rocket or other herbs with the spinach, but use your common sense. We can roll some spinach with a rolling pin, and then cut it up, both for lasagnes and pizzas, which we will make in a little while. This type of sauce is even better. Add the sour cream with a spoon at the very end, so that the texture of the spinach sauce remains compact, as the knives would liquefy the sour cream. Make sure the consistency is right. The spinach sauce is very good with finely chopped garlic and a great bunch of chopped parsley. Various herbs and spices are for different tastes and occasions, but the basis remains the same, without cooking.

This spinach sauce goes well with potatoes, pasta, rice and especially gnocchi. Make the gnocchi according to the classic recipe, just use whole-wheat Kamut flour instead of white. Cook the potatoes, grind, knead with the flour, roll about a thumb thick rolls, slice them and cook in salted boiling water for 20 min. It is not my job to teach classic cooking, which I'm sure most of you know all too well. My job is to point to the finer improvements, which have huge consequences on the health. My goal is to show you how to combine cooked and raw food correctly – the best of both worlds. Good cooking is about good combinations.

When Popeye first heard about this recipe, he quickly tossed away all his cans of spinach and has been using the hand blender ever since. Olive was so impressed that she fainted and loves him more than ever before.

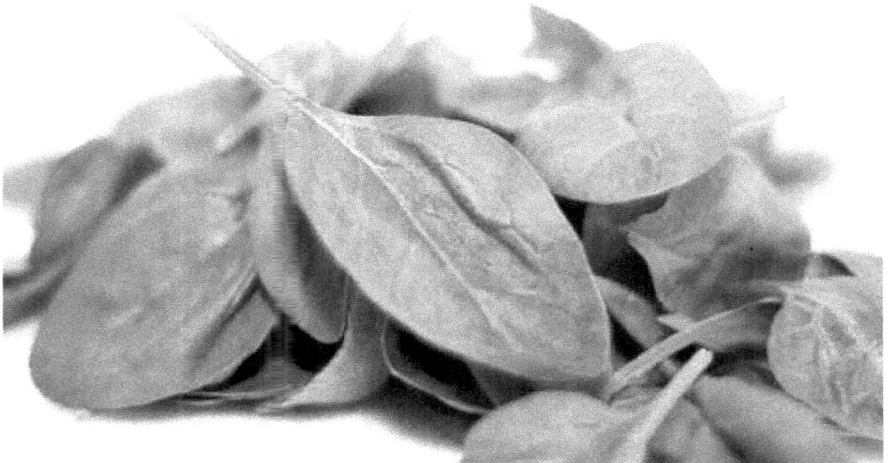

Classic tomato sauce:
500 g ripe organic tomato,
50 g dry tomatoes,
a slice of Hokkaido pumpkin,
6-8 tbs olive oil,
garlic clove,
fresh or dry basil,
oregano,
salt

Tomato chilli sauce:
500 g tomato,
50 g dry tomato,
1 red pepper,
1 ts sweet paprika powder,
chilli pepper,
olive oil,
garlic clove,
salt,
pinch of pepper

Herbal tomato sauce:
500g tomato,
50g dry tomato,
parsley root,
celery stalk or celery root,
6-8 tbs olive oil,
garlic clove,
bunch of parsley leaves,
any herbs,
salt

PASTA WITH TOMATO SAUCE

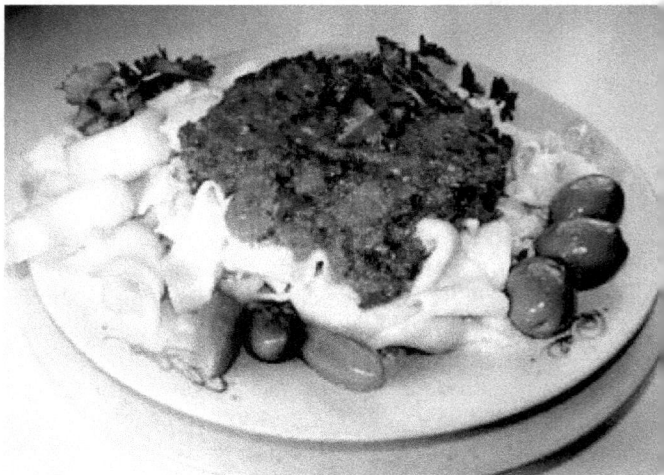

Out of all the sauces the one most consumed is the tomato sauce. Before some 200 years fresh tomato was not eaten in Northern America, because it was falsely believed that it was poisonous. It was eaten only in the form of well-cooked and spiced ketchup. Only a few generations later we now know that cooked tomatoes are in fact toxic. The history of disbeliefs. Conscious scientists warn: after cooking the oxalic acid binds the calcium in the body, which causes arthritis, sclerosis, rheumatism, osteoporosis, cancer, dementia, etc. These are long lists, in fact entire lexicons.

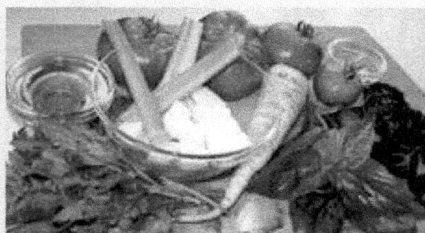
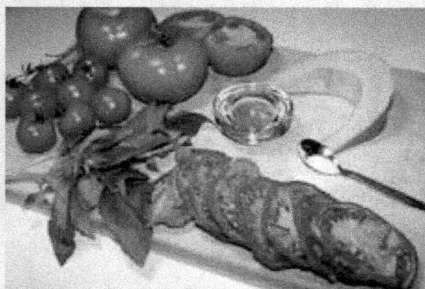
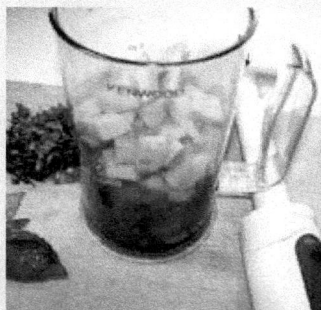
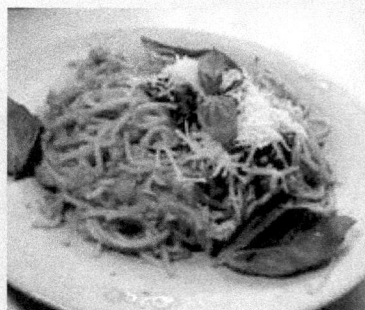

Man made hell out of tomatoes. Step back into paradise, to your ecological garden, where the sauce spends long months cooking in the sun.

The first secret of a good tomato sauce is ripe organic tomato which gives the sauce best texture. Top sauces develop by organic production and ripeness, when the tomato falls into your hands, when it is truly ripe. The second secret is sun-dried tomato, which thickens the sauce and enhances the flavor; chop it up and soak for 10-15 minutes before preparing the sauce. The third secret is Hokkaido pumpkin or red pepper. These two ingredients make the sauce smooth and fine. The fourth secret is in the correct preparation of the chopped vegetables and spices: finely chop the onion, garlic, basil, oregano, parsley leaves like the cooking chefs. The fifth secret is the additions: stewed mushrooms, egg plant cubes and soy meat as a substitute to meat, naturally preserved olive slices and capers for the taste of Mediterranean. The last secret I am goint to reveal to you is Ñame – the root which you can buy only in south America, Canary Islands and tropical and subtropical regions. A slice of Ñame makes sauce smooth and amazingly good tasting.

It's not difficult to make a good sauce out of good ingredients. Mix the fresh tomatoes with a hand blender, Hokkaido pumpkin, peppers, soaked dry tomatoes or the main ingredients from the recipes above, which we chopped already. Add the finely chopped onion, garlic, basil, oregano, parsley leaves, chives, chili, whatever,..., a little traditional virgin olive oil and a tiny teaspoon of salt. Beware – when purchasing olive oil check for mark **cold pressed** on a bottle, because label saying Extra virgin olive oil is misleading... usually it is termically processed and consequently hazardous and ocourse of inferior taste.

The sauces warm up once you pour them over hot pasta. For a touch of Asia, replace a part of pasta with zucchinis, which you can slice to thin strips with a vegetable peeler, then marinate in soy sauce and oil and serve with the pasta. You can prepare pasta like this as an appetizer – or antipasto as the Italians say. If you love Italian cuisine, but are trying to eat healthier, a smaller plate of pasta can be an appetizer, whereas for the main course you can have one of the salads from the plentiful repertoire. Good morning New World!

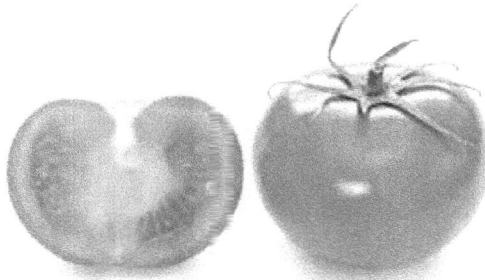

Enriched mashed potatoes:
1 kg potatoes,
smaller celery root 250-400 g,
1.5 dl of sour cream,
50-80 g raw butter from raw milk or
a couple spoons of sunflower oil,
salt

Endless way to enrich the puree:
parsley root,
parsnip,
white turnip...

ENRICHED MASHED POTATOES

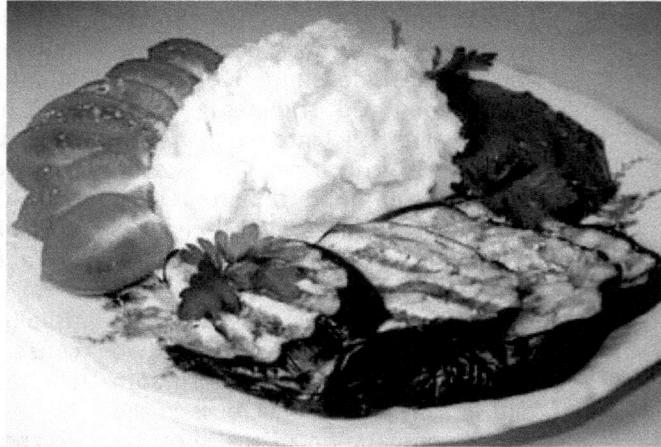

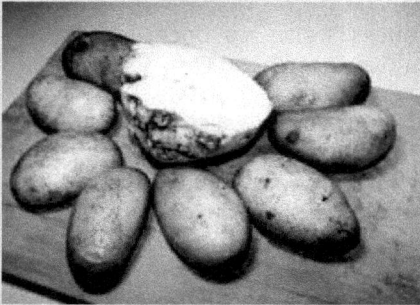

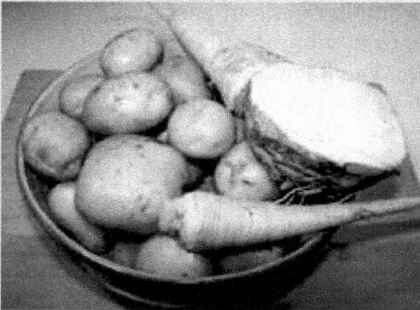

The present recipe will bring joy to those who love a classic lunch and especially mashed potatoes, because they can now make it **in a healthier way**. The secret is in the grated celery root. This is full of natural salts, which naturally enhance the flavor and add freshness to the mashed potatoes. **The positive effects celery has on your body was described by Dr. Norman Walker in the book Fresh Vegetable and Fruit Juices.** Natural organic sodium and calcium are the ones, which are plentiful in celery, which helps the entire nervous system; soothes, relaxes and opens the breath.

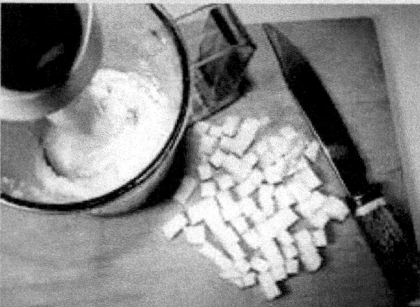
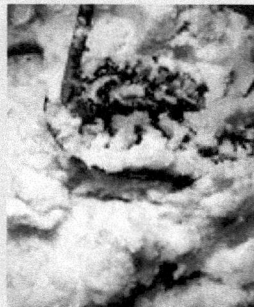
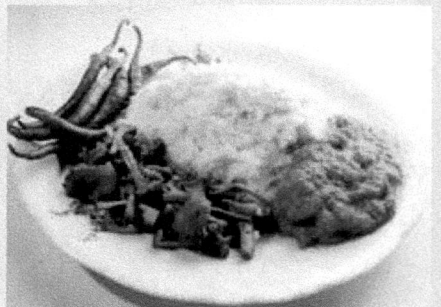

I remember feeling drowsy after normal mashed potatoes. But after having these mashed potatoes you won't feel sleepy like you normally did after a classical lunch, especially if you serve it with spinach or tomato sauce. You will explode from all the vivacity. Why give up a popular dish, if in fact it can even have healing effect?

Cook the potatoes, mash them and wait for them to cool a bit. While the potatoes are cooling, grate the celery, which is somewhat time-consuming, but gives the best results. Or you can chop up the celery and blend it with a hand blender into a puree with a few spoons of oil. The way in which you are going to make celery root into fresh puree depends on the utensils you have at your disposal, but make sure it's as smooth as it can be. Mix the grated celery root, sour cream and pieces of butter into the potato puree, while it's still warm, but not hot, as the heat would destroy the vitamins in the celery and all the qualities of fresh cream and butter. We have to seize the right moment, so that the dish is served warm and the vitamins preserved.

Some people don't like raw vegetables. For them this recipe is an excellent way for their body to get the life important minerals in a way that their taste buds don't get upset because the good old mashed potatoes are still a main part of the dish. A lot of children are growing up on artificial food and candy, but with a small dietetic trick you can change their lives. Start with a small amount of celery in the potatoes and gradually increase the amount. They won't even notice it and their body cells will scream with excitement. Parsley, parsnip and turnip also go well with mashed potatoes if we want to experiment. Also some grilled (without oil) mushrooms, zucchinis or eggplants fit perfectly with the mashed potatoes.

Usually, the first thing a doctor will do is ban all cooked vegetables from a diet, and replace it with fresh. If this is not possible, then he skillfully adds the medicine in the dish. A good doctor is a dietician.

Dr. Norman Walker, one of the pioneers in the area describes celery as one of the most important nutrients in a healthy diet side by side with greens. It should be regularly on the menu but how can we include it in a meal if it does not taste as good on its own? In the next recipe we will describe one of the greatest innovations in dietetics of this century.

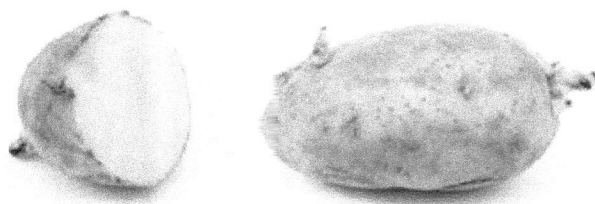

Healing Vegetable Soup

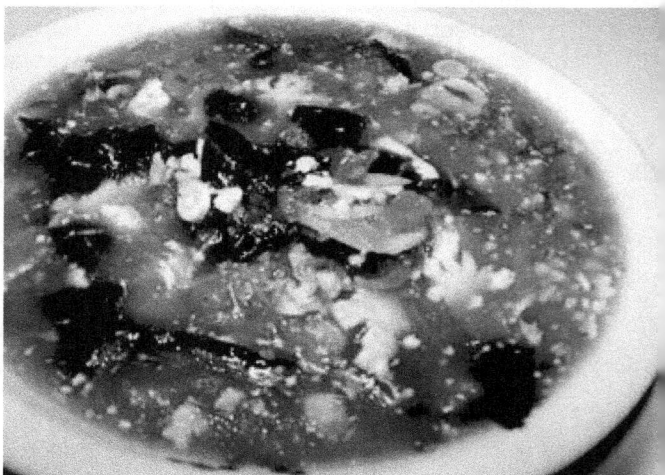

Healing stock:
2-4 peppers,
2-4 cucumbers,
2-4 ripe tomatoes,
1 celery root,
half of celery green

Vegetable for soup:
cauliflower,
broccoli,
aladdin,
smaller carrot,
parsley root and leaves,
20 g of arame algae,
20 g of wakame algae,
5-10 tbs sunflower oil,
½ ts salt,
fresh spices,
100 g grated fresh cheese or
avocado

Vegetable and stock:
parsley leaves,
¼ grated red pepper,
noodles,
broccoli...

Fresh vegetable juices are liquid gold from the viewpoint of health, but only a small number of people enjoy their blessings. I was thinking, how to get more people to enjoy fresh juices and one day it dawned on me: Soups! In fact, I had made my first simple soup a few years before, but only later did I discover the potential it had. I tried recipe after recipe and slowly transformed the juices into soups. A smile crept to my face – this is the solution for widespread use! From the first soup a rich menu of selection was born. Because soups are eaten with spoons and we have to somewhat chew them, the assimilation

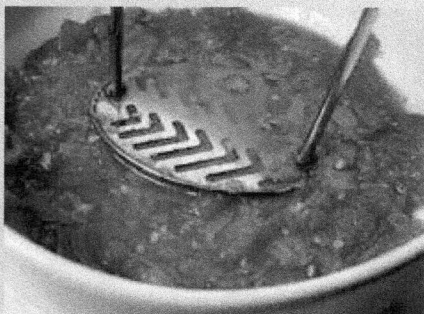

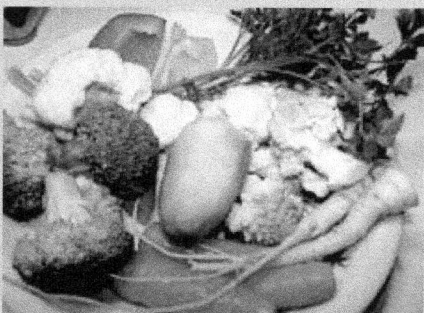

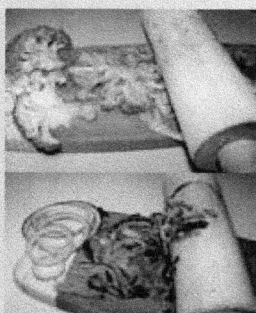

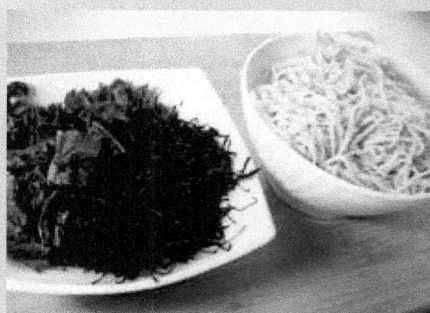

of healing effects is even better than with drinking juices. Since soups are an everyday classic the consequences of this culinary innovation are far-reaching. Each household, house and health institution should have such soups on their daily menus. I even took a step further and dismissed the compulsory equipment – the juicer.

The preparation is simple. Firstly, choose organically grown vegetables which give the soup tender sweet taste, as the ordinary ones bitters it. **Chop up the tomatoes and mash them like potatoes to get pure tomato juice, don't mix it in a blender - squash it by hand. Cut the wakame algae with scissors, crush the arame in your fist and mix in both algae with the mashed tomato to soften.** Squeeze the juice out of peppers, cucumbers and celery with a juicer and pour it in the revolutionary pot. We can also cut up the vegetables and mix in a blender than sift through a strainer. With hand blender is quicker and there is less washing up to do. Finely chop the parsley leaves, cauliflower, broccoli aladdin, a quarter of pepper, finely grate half a carrot and slice of celery to thicken the soup. If algae and grated cheese seem unusual in the soup, we can add noodles to it but we have to cook them separately. In the end, add the cold pressed oil, salt and pepper stir and season according to taste.

One representative of the first generation of natural healers, Dr. Norman Walker managed to prove that the best cure in the world is the vegetable juices. The second generation managed to produce the recipes suitable for everyday use –healing soups. The recipe has only one thing missing – it is not hot when served. Consider this: it is better for the soup to be warm and you to feel warm, than for it to be hot and you cold. Before the preparation keep the vegetables at room temperature and you can also heat up the soup with the stock which you cooked separately. I usualy cook hotchpotch of vegetables that need to be cooked (potato, yuca, peas, beans, chick pea, mushrooms, etc...) blend it a bit to get right texture and serve it hot. By the side of it I serve cold soup based on celery juice (Celery root, celery stalk, carrot, smashed tomato, parsley, etc...) So first you can enjoy hot soup if you like it and when it cools down a bit mix vitamin bomb into the soup – a little trick.

Making the soup will require some more effort but it will be amply repaid as all or most of the enzymes, minerals and vitamins will remain 100% intact. **For a few extra minutes spent on the preparation, you will gain decades more of healthy living. A fair trade!** If we compare a cooked soup with the healing fresh soup is like comparing a ragged beggar with a queen adorned in golden embroidered clothes. Fire makes dead ash out of living gold – reverse alchemy. **Away with fire, there is a revolution on the way to your kitchen.**

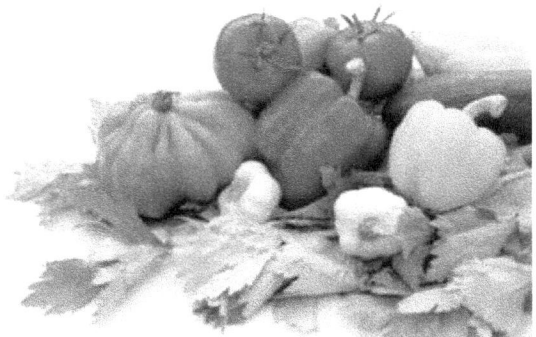

Corn or Kamut tortillas:
250 g Corn or Kamut flour,
water,
salt

Natural ajvar:
2 red peppers,
50 g of dry tomatoes,
½ dl of sunflower oil,
1 ts red pepper,
garlic clove,
chilli,
eggplant optional.

Vegetable for tortillas:
avocado,
different lettuces,
onion,
zucchini,
tomato,
eggplants,
mushrooms,
alfalfa sprouts...

TORTILLA WITH AJVAR

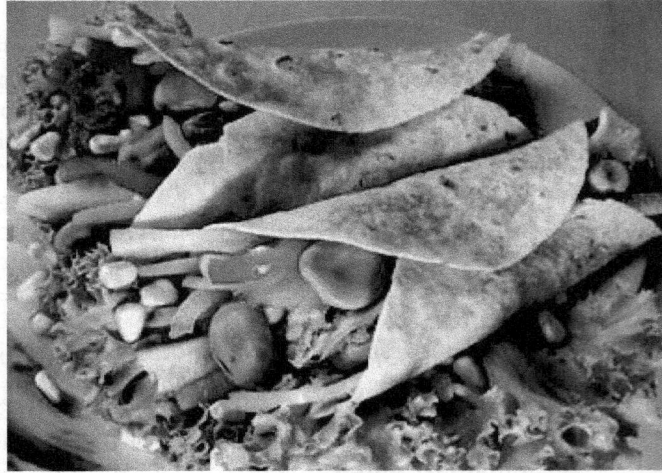

Mexican food has become popular around the world, therefore it has to have an important part in our recipes. This recipe joins two traditional dishes from Southern places: the Southern American tortilla and Ajvar, which originates from the Balkans. The combination might not win over the world, but it can win your hearts. You can buy tortillas in every supermarket, but beware; wheat flour is "junk food". It's best if you bake your own corn or Kamut tortillas. Mix the flour, water, and salt into stiff dough, make the balls, flour them and roll between two sheets of polyvinyl to about 2 mm of

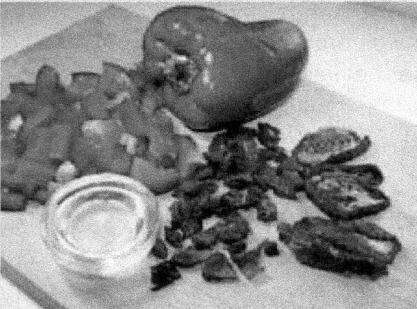
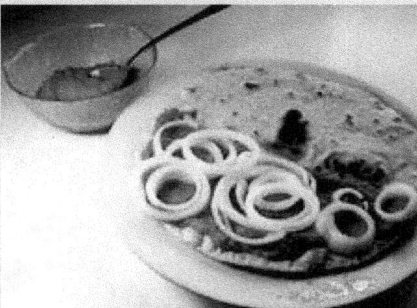
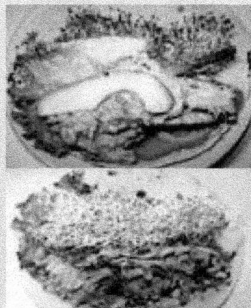
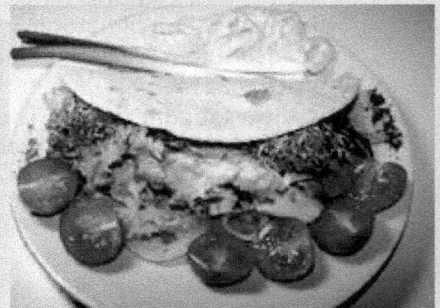

thickness. With a bowl turned upside down, cut out the tortillas of about 20 cm in diameter and bake in a pan without grease for a good minute on both sides. Alternatively, you can find the recipe for tortilla from other sources.

And now is the time for the guest star of the evening - Ajvar. According to the traditional method Ajvar is made by grilling the peppers and eggplants, peeling the peppers, and finally grinding and cooking for long hours in sunflower oil to thicken. In this way vitamins A and C disappear, the oil is ruined and the blood vessels are clogged. Stroke!A million stories.

We will make Ajvar from fresh juicy peppers, cold pressed oil and dry tomatoes which will thicken the Ajvar in minutes and miraculously give it the flavor the same as if we had cooked and grilled it. Cut up the dry tomatoes, soak for about 15 minutes and blend with a hand blender. Add the chopped peppers, red paprika powder, oil and grind once more. For the final texture add some oil at the very end and mix well with a spoon. Some finely chopped garlic and the Balkan specialty will soon join the Southern American. For the flavor of the American South add some chilli.

Those who prefer the original Ajvar variety can grill the eggplants and then thinly cut them and mix them in the specialty. We will stuff the tortillas with the grilled eggplants. Raw eggplants don't taste good and have no particular nutritional value contrary to peppers so we can grill them without worries. We don't need to explain that the taste of natural Ajvar is far superior compared to the cooked one; it is healthier and more flavorsome. Try it! The recipe for Ajvar is not good only for tortillas, originally it is a spread for bread or it can be served as a side dish with vegetable dishes.

Onion rings, lettuce, rocket, slice of avocado, alfalfa sprouts, grilled mushrooms, eggplants, zucchini. Stuff the tortillas as you wish, fold and you will get tacos, as they are called in Mexico. You can put anything in tortillas, but keep it green.

The 21st century is fantastic, you can hop on a plane and travel to the other end of the world or switch the TV channel and you're there. And there's a third option to experience two continents at the same time; join two traditional dishes on a plate.

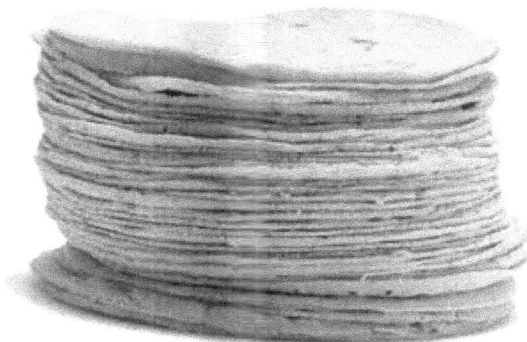

Leek noodles:
½ leek (150 g),
1 zucchini (250 g),
200 g of Kamut noodles

Parmesan cheese sauce:
70-100 g of ripe
goat or lamb cheese,
1 dl of sour cream,
3-4 tbs of sesame or olive oil,
lime juice,
pine nuts,
salt,
white pepper

Smooth cheese sauce:
without pine nuts
+3 tbs of raw butter and garlic clove

LEEK NOODLES IN CHEESE SAUCE

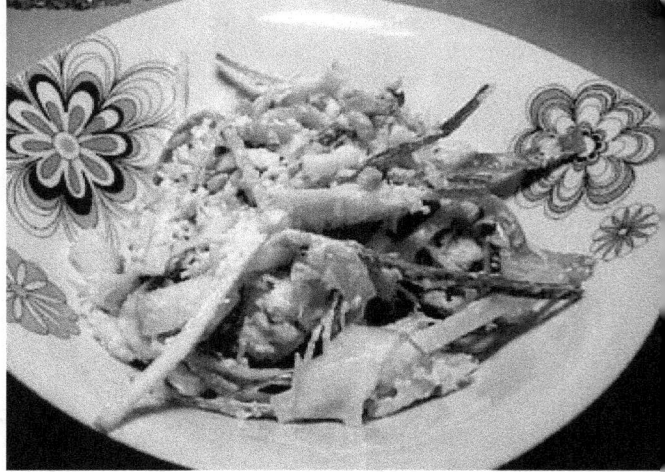

The inspiration for this next dish comes from the Italian and French cuisine. Delicious cheese sauce is the fresh variety of the Hollywood renowned Alfredo sauce, originally from a small restaurant in Rome. Spicy leek and juicy zucchini noodles are according to the French taste, whereas we gourmands round off the worldly romance with a touch of Kamut noodles. All dairy products in this recipe are from raw milk and are currently hard to find. In your nearest dairy store, request that they obtain raw rather than processed variety and insist in your demand, as pasteurization will sooner or later seize to

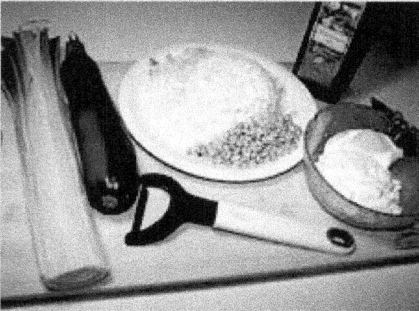

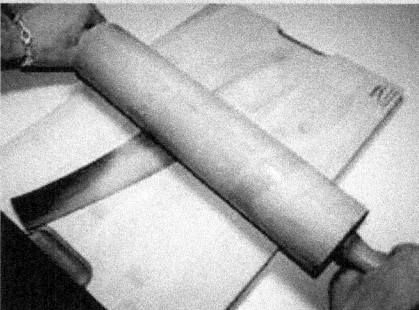

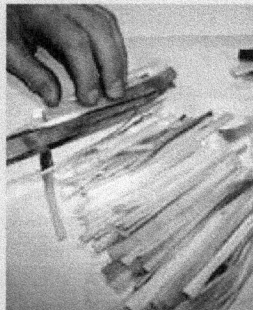

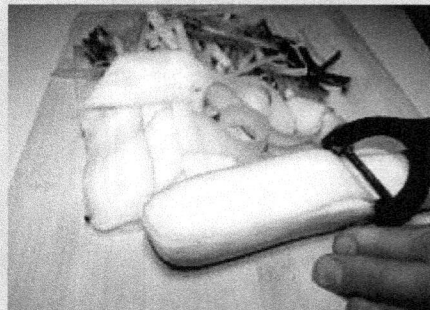

exist – it will be banished.

Rinse the leek and roll each leaf with a roller to squeeze the juice out. Slice the leaves into stripes, first the stalk into thirds, then into thin noodles. With a vegetable peeler, slice the zucchini into thin leaves and in half to get wide zucchini noodles. The spicy mixture of leek and zucchini noodles can be served as an independent dish. You can also cook the Kamut noodles; just cool them a bit before mixing in with the spicy ones.

The first cheese sauce is grainy thanks to texture of grated cheese. Grate the cheese and mix in the sour cream, sesame oil, pinch of white pepper, some drops of lime juice, salt, stir well with the spicy noodles and sprinkle the pine nuts on top. **The taste is romantic, French and somewhat spicy.** If leek taste is too strong add some yellow salad leaves.

The other cheese sauce is creamy. In a double bowl, melt the raw butter, just make sure that the water in the bottom bowl is not hot, just warm. Blend sour cream, grated cheese and melted raw butter in a mixer. Crush the garlic clove with some spoons of oil in a mortar and add the mixture into the sauce. The sauce is greasy but very delicious. **Pour it over the elegant combination of noodles, light the candles and put on some classical music.**

The well-known fact that we should avoid greasy food is a half-truth, or let's say a lesser important part of the truth. The more important part of the warning is the quality of fat. High temperature spoils the fat, instead of long chains, only cringed up spirals remain, botches and clogs. The Nobel prize for pasteurization awarded in the previous century was a mistake, which the today's generation should correct.

Since raw dairy products are hard to obtain in large cities, many people opt for vegan food. The dairy industry and distribution of dairy products should be reorganized. Let's hope that the good old times come back soon, when there will be a bottle of milk waiting for you in the morning in front of your door, a slice of real cheese and real raw butter with a milkman waving goodbye at you on his bike as he goes on his way. I heard that in some parts of Britain the good old practice continues... Oh, world unite in good practices.

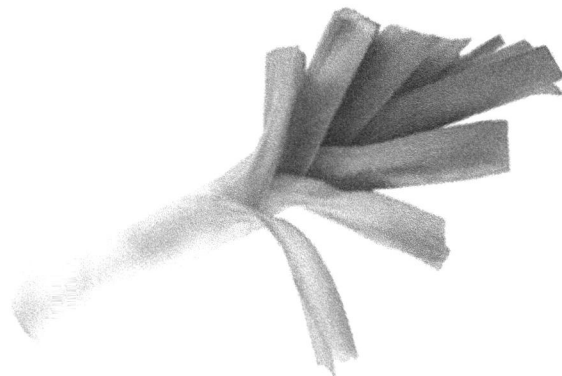

French salad:
800 g potatoes,
400 g peas,
500 g naturally conserved pickles,
300 g carrots,
100 g soya beans for those,
who wish to replace eggs

Natural mayonnaise:
150 g sunflower seeds,
juice of one lemon,
cup of water,
2 dl of sunflower oil,
1/4 ts of salt

FRENCH SALAD

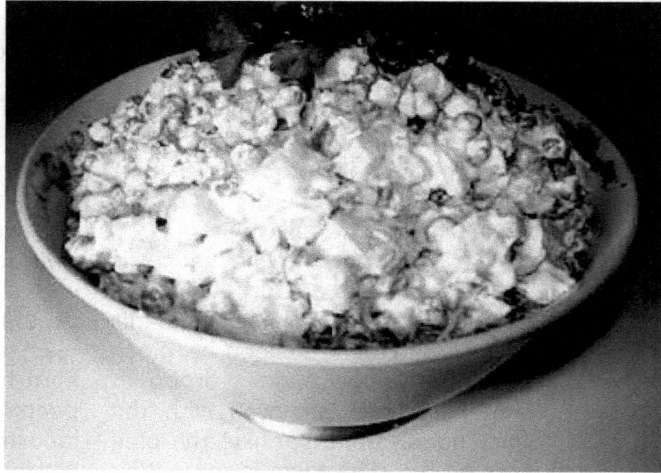

In Slovenia and Crotatia we know it as French salad, in France it's called Russian salad or "Salad Russe", in Russia Oliver's salad after a Moscow inventor. It is a mess, but a very good salad indeed. Let's explore some more. **The French adopted it from the Russians and named it Russian salad. Since the vegetables are chopped up in French style and the mayonnaise is French, some call it French salad.** More than a salad, it soon became a festive dish, served especially for Christmas and New Year parties. According to our philosophy, we will make it in a much healthier way. Oliver would love it!

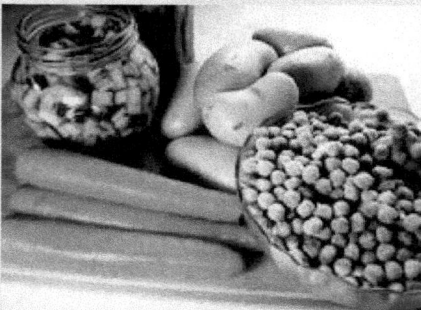

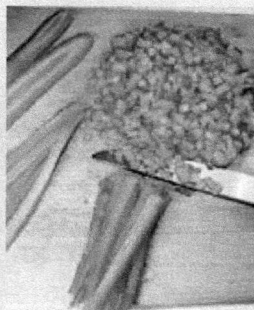

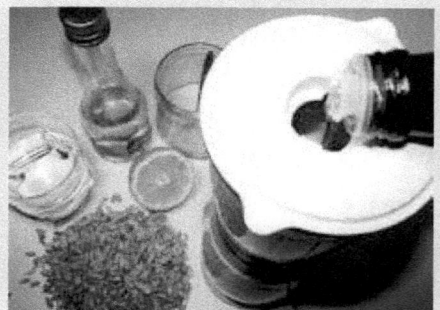

Conserve the pickles at least a day or two before you begin preparing the salad. Slice them to about a centimeter thick sticks, fill a glass jar and pour over a mixture of water, vinegar and spices. Add about 3.5 dl of apple vinegar, cumin, black pepper and a garlic clove to 7dl of water. Read more about natural conservation in recipe 34.

In classic mayonnaise there is a bunch of eggs, a burden for the kidneys and liters of motor oil, as I call refined oil. Natural mayonnaise is far superior and made in such a simple way that it's hard to believe. Brilliant simplicity achieved with natural ingredients. Let's get to it.

Mix the sunflower seeds with a cup of water in a blender. Leave for a minute or two to bloat, squeeze the lemon, add the juice, ½ ts of salt until the mixture is smooth and thick, then begin to slowly add the cold pressed sunflower oil. Add the oil in a thin stream for at least half a minute or longer for the cream to

really foam up into mayonnaise. We add the oil slowly, otherwise it won't become mayonnaise. Gourmets can replace one half of sunflower seeds with pine nuts.

Cook the potatoes, peel and cut them up into about a centimeter cubes. Cook the peas separately and mix them in with the potatoes (If you have young sweet peas you don't need to cook them as they are soft and delicious). Cut the pickles into about a centimeter cubes. **Do not cook the carrots, just cut them into cubes about 6-7 mm, smaller than usually cooked carrots.** Cooking nutrients full of vitamins is one of the greatest mistakes in the culinary world. **Why cook the carrots? Make the cubes smaller and the salad becomes crunchier and full of vitamin A.** Pour over the mayonnaise, stir and serve. We saved 75% of ingredients from destructive power of fire. Imagine Moscow in front of you and white snowflakes.

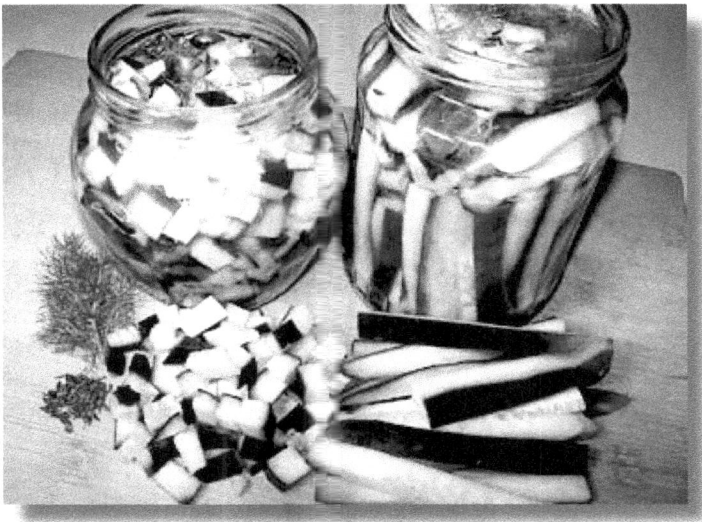

Super pate:
100 g sunflower seeds,
0.75 dl water,
juice of one lemon,
salt or soy sauce,
1.5 dl of sunflower oil,
100 g tofu

Super spreads:
Super pâté and the ingredients
according to the recipes below

SUPER PÂTÉ AND SUPER SPREADS

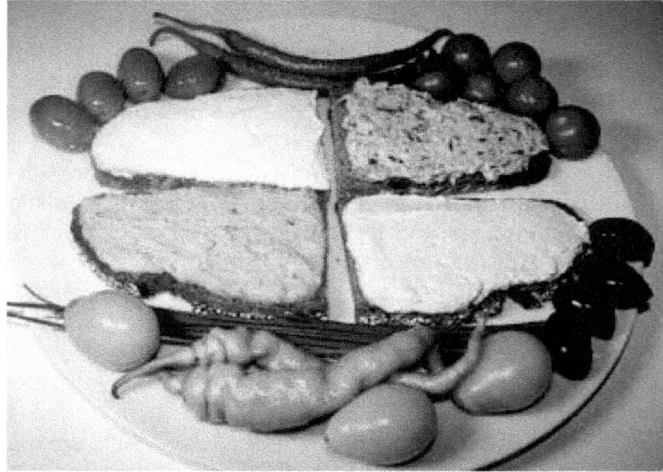

If you knew what is in your ordinary pâtés, you would never buy them again. If you knew super pâtés, you wouldn't wish for any other. If you knew the secret of preparation, you would make them again and again. If only you knew how good they are, each in its own way....

We'll make the super pâté in a similar way to the mayonnaise for the French salad. The only difference is that we will add less water to the sunflower seeds in the blender. When the blades start to spin, add it with a spoon through the opening on top. The mixture should

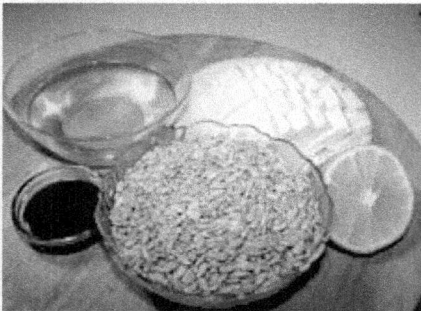

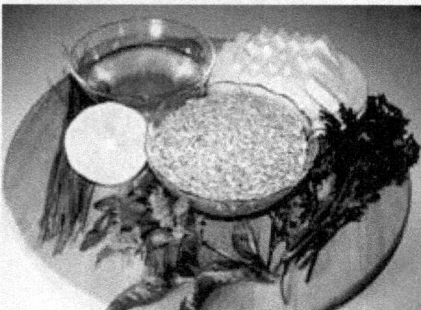

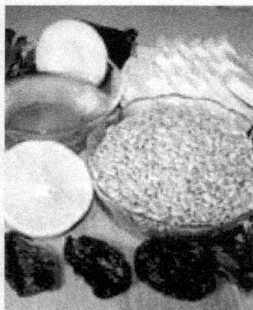

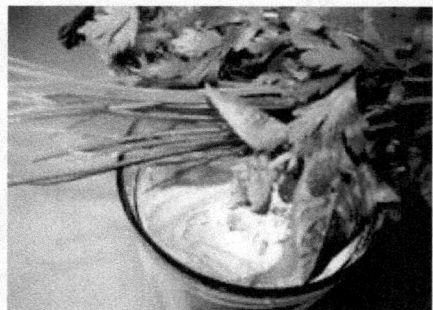

be thick for it to barely spin. Then begin to add the oil in a thin stream. When it becomes thick, add the tofu cubes and spin some more. Try different tofu's and cold pressed oils. If you want original chicken pâté, use soy sauce instead of salt. Great! To turn the pâté into a spread you just add spices, herbs and vegetables.

Vegetable spreads with 10-12% herbs are not real herbal spreads. Herbal super spreads contain 25-50% herbs. They may include a large bunch of parsley leaves, the green leaves of a young onion, bunch of fresh basil, oregano, chives - basically any fresh spices or herbs available. finely chop them up and mix in a blender with the pâté for a few seconds to release the juice in order to soak and flavor the spread. Yummy!

We get the super vegetable spread by adding 3-4 halves of dry tomatoes, ¼ of red pepper, ½ onion, ¼ smaller zucchini and 1 ts of red paprika powder. Finely chop the vegetables and blend them with the basic ingredients. For the spicy version, add some chilli and pepper. Hot!

For horse-radish super spread first naturally conserve the horse-radish. Grate the horse-radish and place in the freezer for an hour to lose its strength. Pour over the juice of two lemons; add a topped teaspoon of salt and mix. Fill a glass jar and pour some oil over it. Naturally conserved horse-radish will stay in the fridge for several months. If we mix in the basic recipe 2-3 tbs of horse-radish, we get the horse-radish super spread.

Wild garlic super spread is the freshness of the forest on your table. In the spring, on the outskirts of the woods, gather the wild garlic and clean it, but never rinse with water. Blend it into a puree with olive oil, ground hazelnuts, walnuts or sunflowers with a hand blender. To about 100 g of mixture add 20 g of hazelnuts, 1 dl olive oil, some tablespoons of lemon juice and salt. Naturally conserved wild garlic will last in the fridge for a couple of weeks, maybe months, depends on hygiene of preparation. If you mix in some spoons of wild garlic into the basic recipe and add a bunch of parsley leaves or basil, you get the wild garlic super spread.

Spreads are especially good on bread made from Kamut and buckwheat flour in the ratio 80:20, because buckwheat is rich with protein and goes well with high protein spreads. Still worried about proteins?

A long long time ago three little dinosaurs tore away the palm leaves as though it was parsley and chatted about the prehistoric myth – the protein myth and laughed. Out of the bushes came the fourth dinosaur and they couldn't hold it much longer, they started laughing, rolling on the grass and banged their 20-meter-tails on the floor, so that the earth shook and the valley resonated with: ha-ha-ha-ha- ho-ho-ho-ho-ho-ho.

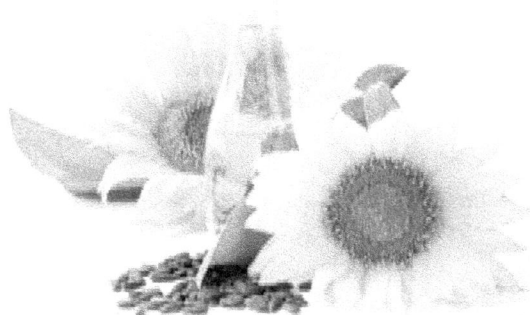

Vegetable risotto:
500 g paddy rice,
400 g frozen peas,
250 g Hokkaido pumpkin,
400 g tomatoes,
1 pepper,
½ smaller leek,
2 carrots,
1 parsley root with leaves,
40 g dry tomatoes,
1 ts of sweet red paprika,
5-7 tbs olive oil,
1 garlic clove,
soy sauce,
curry.

Butter risotto:
500g rice,
250g shitake mushrooms or
champignons or both,
200g frozen peas
(or 100 g of deshelled hemp seeds),
1 zucchini,
¼ broccoli,
1 smaller pumpkin,
½ onion,
50g raw butter made of fresh milk,
6-7tbs coconut oil,
4 artichokes,
parsley leaves,
garlic clove,
pinch of white pepper,
salt

VEGETABLE AND BUTTER RISOTTO

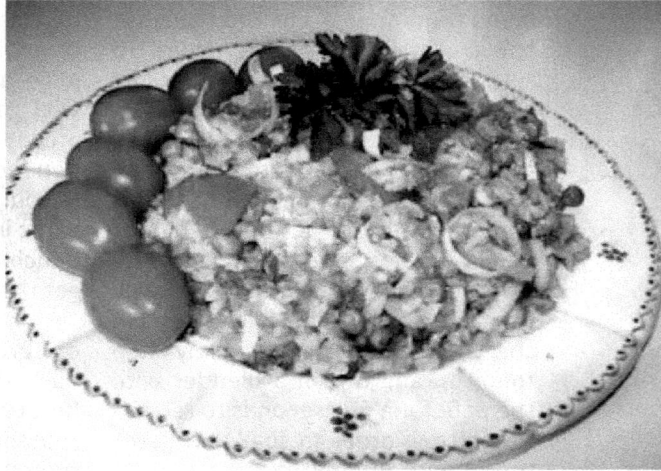

Risotto is one of the top 10 most popular dishes in the world. Did you know that rice is the staple food for some two thirds of the world population? Recipes for risotto differ, each chef has its own, but from every recipe we can make a healthy version if we stick to the basic principle: cook, braise and grill only the ingredients which are not edible raw such as rice, peas, mushrooms and eggplants. All other ingredients should be mixed in natural state in an appropriate way: tomatoes, peppers, carrots, leek, parsley, etc... I will demonstrate this principle with my recipe. I hope that you will like it and

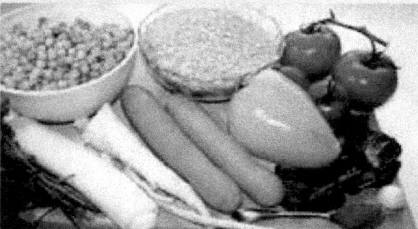

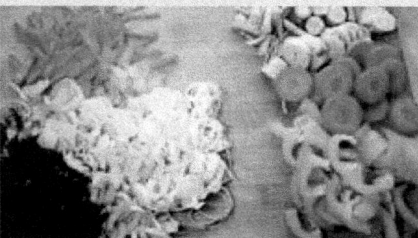

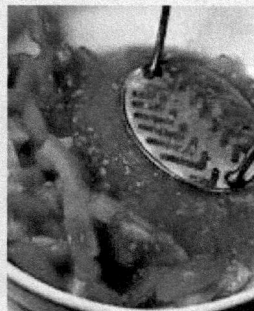

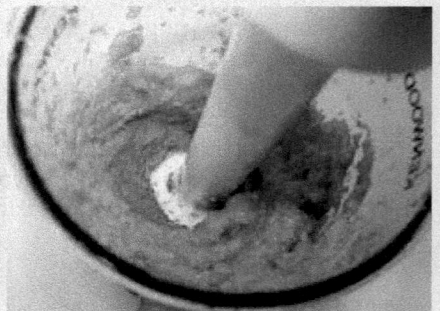

that it will inspire you to **create new recipes or adapt the ones you use.**
Cook the peas in a liter and a half of water for 10 minutes, then add the Hokkaido pumpkin sliced into cubes and cook for another 15 minutes. In a low bowl, sauté the rice on a moderate fire without grease for 5-7 minutes and constantly stir with a wooden spoon. With the stock from the peas and pumpkin water the rice slowly i.e. steam it by adding a ladle of soup occasionally, frequently checking the taste. In the meanwhile prepare the fresh vegetables.

Cut up the tomatoes and mash it so that it resembles braised tomatoes. Leek with its special flavor in combination with soy sauce replaces the grilled onion. Chop it up into thin slices. Cut half of pepper into tiny cubes and a small carrot into tiny sticks. We can also use a mandolin for the carrot sticks. If we prefer onion, we can grill only half of it and chop the other half into the risotto raw to preserve some of its healing nutrients.

We have chopped up some of the vegetables. Some we will blend into a sauce: the larger carrot, parsley root, half of pepper, 1 ts of red paprika powder, soy sauce olive oil and soaked dry tomato Chop the parsley leaves and garlic Then mix the vegetables, rice, peas and Hokkaido pumpkin mix into a glorious, healthy risotto. Usually after

risotto is cooked we wait for a couple of minutes to cool down and than mix it with the raw ingredients.We will have to acquire some experience to catch the right moment, when the risotto is warm enough to serve, but the vitamins in the vegetables still intact by heat.

Butter risotto is similar to seafood risotto. Sauté the rice for a couple of minutes without grease, add the shitake mushrooms, pour over hot water and in the end add the peas. Artichokes you don't need to cook, just cut stalks and a few leaves away, than cut one inch top and slice into thin slices. You can pickle raw artichokes in cold pressed olive oil a few days before. Mix the rice into a bigger bowl and stir here and there for it to cool down faster. When it gets to the right temperature, add the finely grated zucchini, chopped onions, garlic, parsley, pieces of raw butter, coconut oil and stir. Serve the rice with the artichoke slices on top and sprinkle some hemp seeds around the artichokes. The starter is another original, cooked artichoke leaves (the hard leaves we peel of before getting to the soft heart) with Alfredo sauce from recipe no. 8. Eat the delicious sauce with the leaves and scrape it with the soft flesh of the artichokes. Perhaps you enjoy the Japanese style rice – "Nori rolls" – you will find the recipe online.

1000 g ripe tomatoes,
600 g peppers (red and green),
150 g alfalfa sprouts,
germinated for 3-4 days
(with green leaves),
½ celery root,
½ celery stalk,
1/2 onion,
150 g white cheese -
goat's or sheep
(for vegans avocado or noodles), 5-6
tbs olive oil,
basil,
oregano,
parsley leaves,
Himalayan salt

HEALING TOMATO SOUP

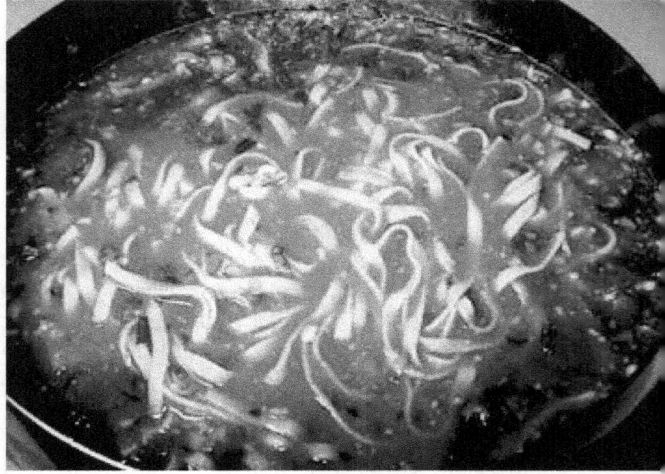

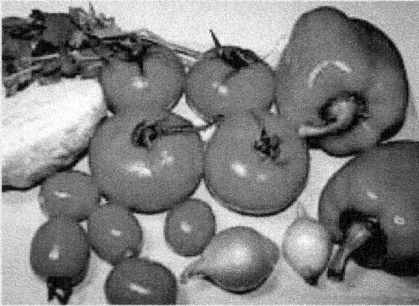

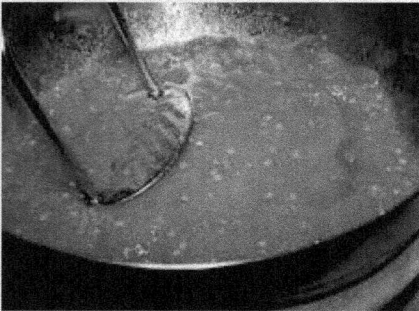

Hippocrates said the most important words in medical history: "Let the food be your medicine and your medicine food." In this recipe we will combine medicine and gastronomy and winn a gold medal. Freshly squeezed juice from baby alfalfa sprouts and celery is one of the best medicines ever discovered. Sprouts carry the youthful energy; the energy of growth; the Indians would call it the energy of spring. The juice from alfalfa sprouts is the same for the renewal of the body and its rejuvenation like the spring sun for vegetation. Celery juice is a rich mixture of organic sodium and

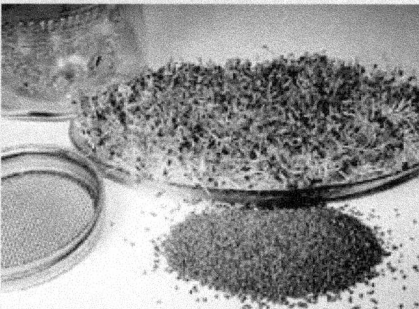

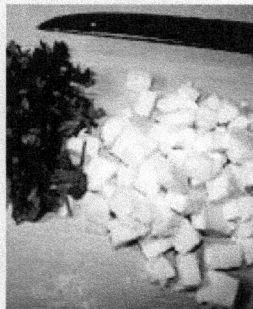

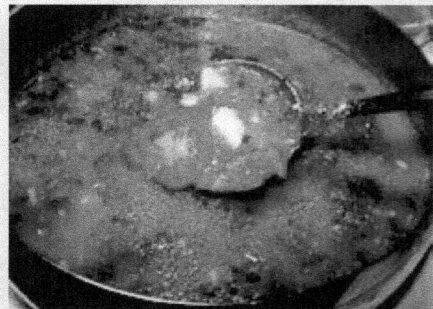

calcium – elements which make the living cells alive. **It is unusual that a medicine tastes as good as this one. The stock from fresh vegetable juices brings tomato soup to the very peak of culinary specialties.** Let's move from medicine to cooking.

First thing first, choose organic vegetables, otherwise the taste will not be right. Chop up the tomatoes, salt and mash into purée. It's faster with a blender, but unprofessional. We don't want a dull texture; we want the pieces of tomato in clear juice. For the juicing of other vegetables we need a juicer. The best ones on the market are Green Star, Omega and Jupiter. Also a blender and strainer can be used. It's easier with a blender, because we only have to chop up the vegetables and the pulp is on the strainer with the juice flowing in under a minute. Cut and juice the peppers, celery, alfalfa sprouts and onion, but be careful with the onion – only add the amount to get some flavor. Pour the juice over the mashed tomato and add spices. Any fresh spices available are good, only make sure you finely chop them. Cut up the cheese, add

some virgin olive oil to the soup and finely stir the ingredients with a ladle. If you prefer creamy tomato soup, blend a ladle of clear soup with half of avocado in a separate bowl, then pour it into the clear soup to thicken it. Soy sauce, pepper, Tabasco or chili are always an option. Tomato soup lovers, get your plates ready.

The first time the taste will be different to what you're used to, but once you get used to it, you won't even consider cooking tomato soup again. Experiment with different vegetables for the stock. Also buckwheat and broccoli sprouts go well with this soup. **To replace** the cheese you can use pieces of whole-wheat bread or separately cook the noodles and add them into soup which will warm up a delicious tomato soup; the healing capacity of the soup remains more or less the same.

After eating healing soup you will feel refreshed, your head will be clear, you will feel relaxed, enjoy a good sleep and this sense of well-being will continue into the following day. The green effects are far-reaching. Please spread the word about this medicinal recipe.

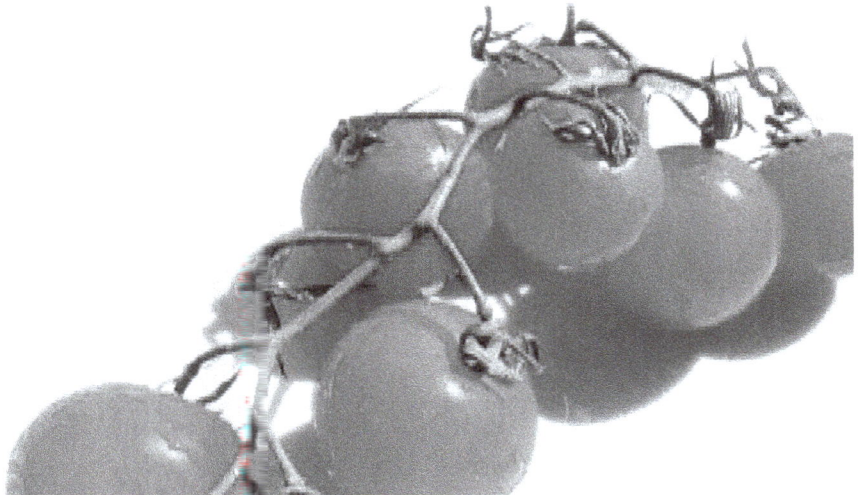

Fresh fruit compotes:
apples and pears

Dry fruit compotes:
Dry fruit,
filtered water,
honey,
agave nectar,
lemon juice,
fresh balm,
mint,
powdered vanilla

NATURAL COMPOTES AND REVITALIZED WATER

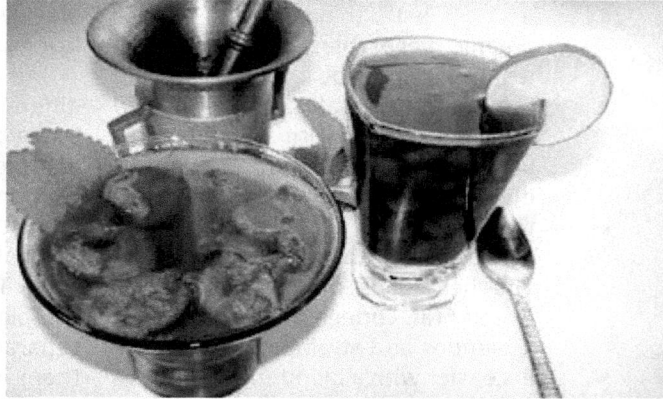

This recipe has the potential to change the entire industry of compotes. Currently this is a dream, but dreams can become reality. Perhaps it seems impossible at first glance, but all that is needed is one small step – a shift in the consciousness of humankind, everything else is fairy tale.

Plentiful baskets of paradise fruit are waiting to be destroyed in fire with kilograms of destructive white sugar added. No! No! **Plentiful baskets of paradise fruit are waiting to be dried slowly in driers and than mixed with paradise honey from beehives on the**

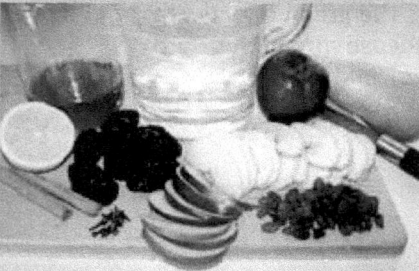

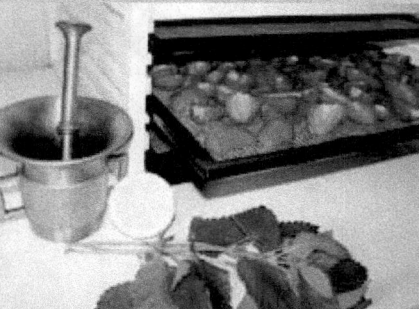

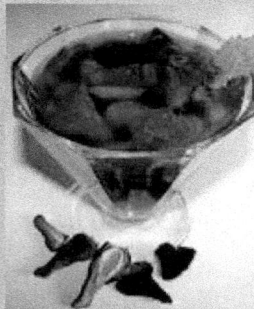

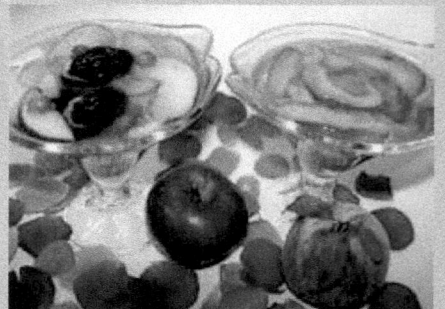

outskirts of orchards. Even the bees will get their honey, half of what they have produced, because they also don't deserve the white death.

Why cook the compotes? When cooking, the vegetable cells in a short period of time crack and release the fluid with all the ingredients to the water, but these ingredients have no life left in them, the temperature boils them. If we slice the apples or pears 3-4 mm thick (no thicker), simply pour over water and leave overnight to soak and the slices will soften like being cooked with the difference that the compote's liquid is 100% living. Here's the recipe: 1.5 l water, 2 soft apples or 2 pears, 5-6 prunes, a handful of raisins, the juice of 1 lemon, 2 spoons of honey, cinnamon and cloves. Keep the glass jar in winter regularly in use.

Apart from apple and pear, most compotes are made from dried fruit. Strawberries, cherries, apricots and prunes are dried in the shape of halves; peaches, pears and larger fruit in slices, cubes, pieces. We dry the fruit at 42ºC for 24-48 hours, or until completely dry. Place it in jars and keep cool for the winter days. When we, for example, want strawberry compote, soak the strawberry halves for 12-24 hours, add lemon or even better lime juice, a tea spoon of agave nectar or honey and the compote is ready made. Another master move for the gourmands: beat juice released from soaked fruit and some balm -mint in a mortar, sift into the compote and the flavor will be unforgettable. Try also real vanilla pod.

There is a lot of talk about water invigoration with commercia products for revitalization, but we **should let Mother Nature do her work. Natural compote changes the energy composition of water. Water becomes charged with negative ions, its life potential increases, and it becomes 'alive'. The surface tension lowers, the water molecules gather into smaller clusters and because of this the water penetrates easier into the body cells.** Water researchers and biologists share the opinion that it is not really about the quantity of water we drink, but the quality of it. The practical use of scientific findings is represented in our famous recipe no. 13. Also make sure to check out the film at **http://www.enwaterment.com/index.php.**

"Come right in" shouts the cell gatekeeper and the gates open, then turns his head and shouts: "Refreshment is heeereee!" All the tiny cell organelles leap with joy and bring out their colorful straws... Natural compote is a very good drink, a kind of cocktail made of physiological solution, which the body cells recognize as their own and immediately release it through the cell membrane, because this is precious 'biological' cargo and refreshment – hydration of cells.

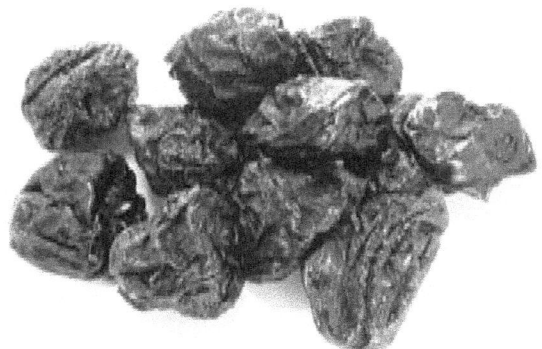

The ingredients are in the text.

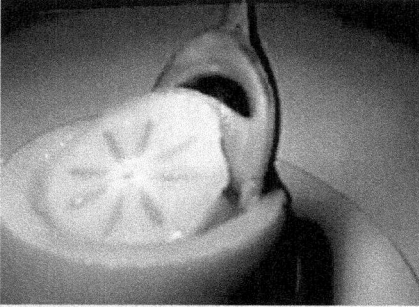

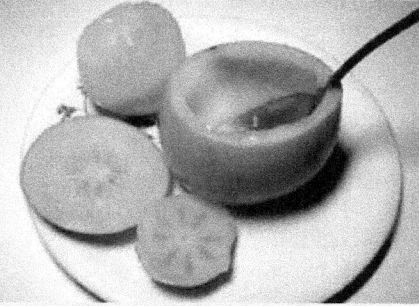

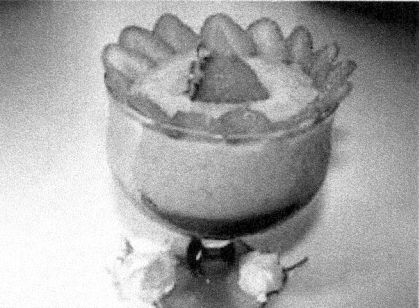

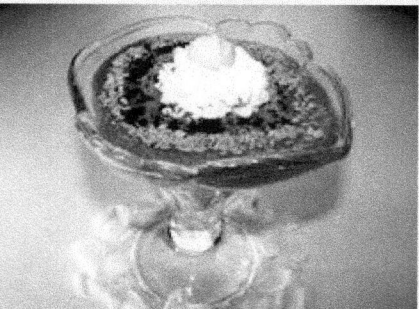

PUDDINGS AND VANILLA CREAM

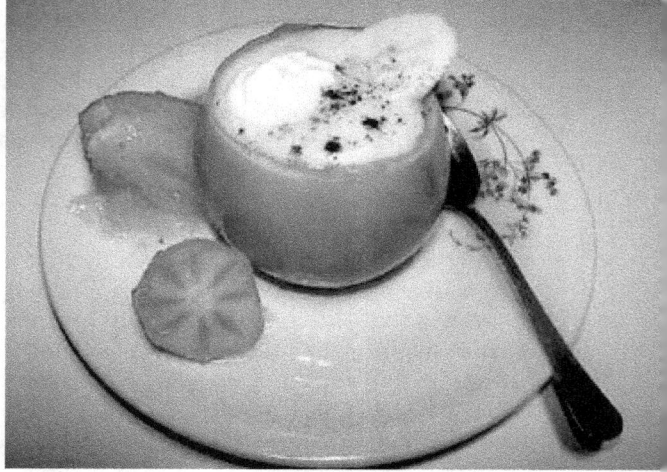

Risalamande in Denmark, budino di riso in Italy, mlečni riž in Slovenia, arroz con leche in Spain and South America, riz au lait in France, rice pudding in America and England, sutlija in Bosnia, kheer in India, riz bi haleeb in Lebanon, ris a la malta in Sweden, riskrem in Norway, khao niao mamuang in Thailand, milchreis in Germany, orez na vareniku in Montenegro, lapa in Macedonia, m'halbi in Africa...etc. As many names, as many different desserts, but the three main ingredients remain the same: rice, milk and sugar.

We won't even talk about

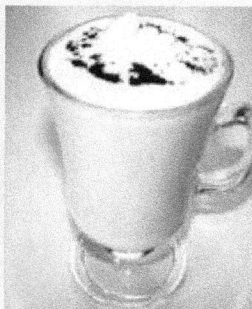

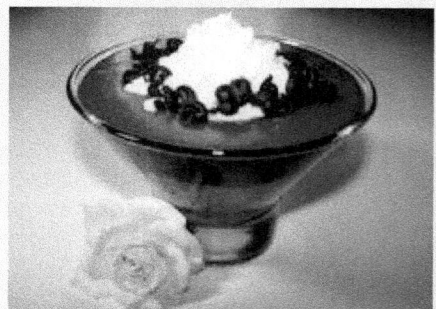

industrial pudding powders; I will simply show you how to make healthy homemade pudding. Whether you sprinkle some orange peel on top like they do it in Italy or add in raisins soaked in rum like in Mexico is a matter of taste and your tradition.

Don't cook the milk, boil the rice on water. Cook it a bit longer than usual. Combine a bowl of cooled rice, a cup of homemade, fresh milk and a spoon of honey or some date nuts in a blender. This is the pudding's base, now select the fruit according to your taste. For silky smooth pudding mix it at maximum power, if you prefer it coarse, mix it less. Some like to add whole cooked rice grains, I myself also like it. So, we got rid of the cooked milk and sugar and are on our way with our makeover and heavenly dessert. A pinch of vanilla and we are in heaven. For chocolate heaven, a topped spoon of powdered cocoa dates a few spoons of cream and a chunk of cocoa butter to make the flavoring genuine.

Cream puddings are even better. Like strawberry for example parboiled rice, soaked dry strawberries sweet cream and agave nectar mixed will take you to seventh heaven. With fresh strawberries we can reach even higher. The amounts are optional a cup of strawberries, a cup of rice and a cup of cream for orientation. **Ecstasy!** Is raspberry, blueberry, peach or apricot pudding still a question? **Now, could you find your own recipe for a raspberry, blueberry, peach or apricot pudding?** The formula is always the same: cooked rice+ fruit or nuts + sweetener + natural fat. For hazelnut pudding grind the hazelnuts mix in some sweet cream to make it super smooth and finally add rice honey and vanilla.

A fantastic **vegan pudding** you get blending 4 bananas, 3-4 topped coconut oil spoons, 2 cups of rice, some dates and powdered vanilla. By the way, this dessert is made in Cambodia.

You have to try **tropical fresh pudding**, if you can get your hands on green coconut. Blend coconut water and soft flesh of two coconuts in a blender, add 4 bananas, powdered vanilla and 70 g of melted fresh cocoa butter. **You are in for an exotic paradise.**

100 % raw pudding with flax is the fastest and healthiest. Flax seeds are a super food, rich in omega 3 fats and roughage. Grind them in a coffee mill and blend in a blender with 4 bananas, 3 topped coconut oil spoons, a spoon of honey a few dates and powdered vanilla. For vanilla pudding, use golden flax, for chocolate brown flax. **Flax gels and puffs up similarly as rice, from a medical point of view this is the healthiest pudding, the best dessert for children and adults.** In a couple of hours in a refrigerator it hardens and forms a crust, like cooked pudding. You can get fresh vegan cream to top it, if you chop up 50 g of macadamia and 20g of truly raw cashews and mix it with some water in a blender, 4 tbs of coconut oil, pinch of vanilla and half a teaspoon of honey.

Vanilla cream is another story. In less than two minutes you will get everything you want. Mix two deciliters of homemade sour cream, 4 bananas and ¼ ts of powdered vanilla in a blender and serve. Only three ingredients but delicious result – the best recipies are simple and delicious; simply delicious. Decorate the puddings according to your mood and desires.

Sprout wafers:
300g Kamut grains,
2 tbs honey,
1 cup of water,
salt

Hazelnut cream:
80g hazelnuts,
60g coconut oil,
2 tbs honey,
½ tbs powdered vanilla

Chocolate cream:
30g hazelnuts,
60g coconut oil,
2 tbs honey,
2-3 tbs powdered cocoa

HAZELNUT AND CHOCOLATE WAFERS

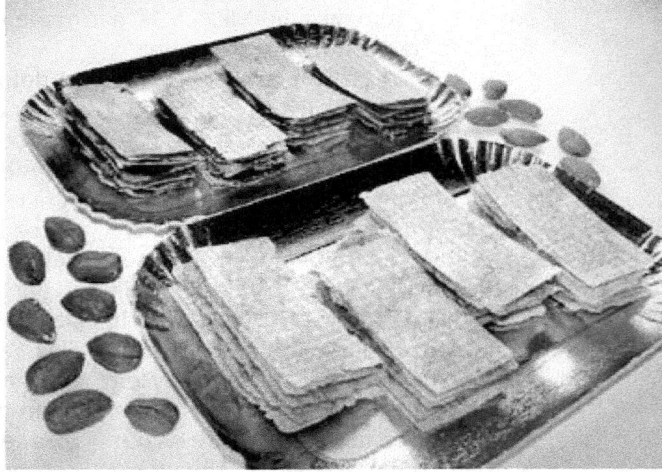

Napoleon would have fought for such a thing. And why not, since it's so good, healthy and made completely without the use of fire. It sounds impossible. I'll let you in on the strategic plan. Take the time to conquer new territory.

First train the army of Kamut grains, germinate them in a glass jar and rinse twice a day. If training is proper with morning and evening shower exactly after 48 hours Kamut is ready for action. Mix a cup of water, sprouts, honey and salt in a blender to medium smooth.

For the wafers we need

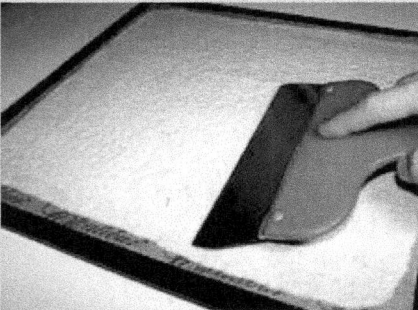
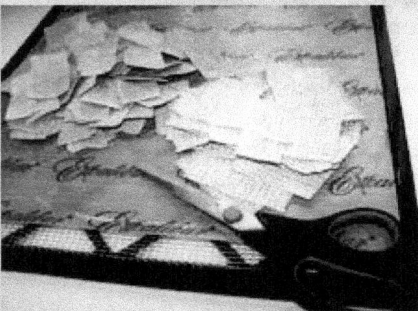
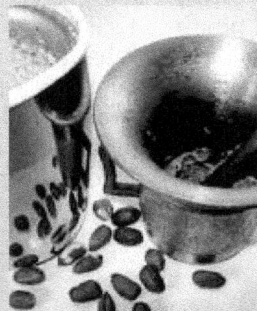
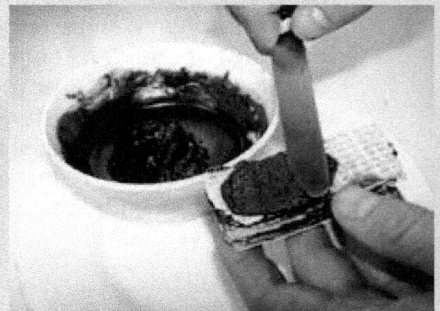

some equipment. Fruit drier and confectionery's spatulas are indispensable. **If you're serious about your health, you will get the drier sooner or later, if for no other reason for the marmalades and compotes, but you can use it for much more than that.** I use Excalibur, but there are many good driers on the market just **avoid the cheap junk**, where you can't accurately regulate the temperature.

Well-equipped we proceed with our operation. With a spoon place the Kamut batter to the drying surface teflex and with a spatula distribute it on the tray in a thin layer When I say thin, I mean pretty thin credit card width thin. This part of the process requires skill and experience the wafers need to be thin, so that they are crunchy and crispy. We will dry them for 3-5 hours at 42ºC Before we place the trays in a drier place a net, which is normally the lining of each drying tray, on top of the thinly layered Kamut batter. With the net, we get the typical structure of wafers and the wafers won't roll up which normally occurs during drying thin layers (remember tree leaves in autumn). When we are fighting for a good cause, certain tricks are allowed. Don't worry if the wafer is too thick the first time, you can use it for apple strudel, which needs thicker layer. If you prefer ordinary baked wafers, you can get them in any supermarket, but go for whole-wheat ones without additives and without sugar – mission impossible at the moment.

Hazelnut cream is a good example of how the simplest thing is best. There are only four ingredients which merge together into complete harmony. Grind the hazelnuts in a coffee mill and mix in coconut oil, honey and vanilla. If you use powdered cocoa and reduce the amount of hazelnuts you will get chocolate cream. Did you expect something more complicated? I tell you, chefs who spent long hours cooking over a moderate flame don't have the faintest idea about gastronomy or healthy cuisine. We are done with them.

Once the wafers are dry, remove them from the drier, cut them up and let's make rafts to get to the other side. We cut the wafers at 3 times 8 cm. We will need scissors; you never know what comes in handy on this mission. Fold the wafers: spread the cream, cover with a wafer, cream, wafer, cream, wafer for 5-7 layers. 30 minutes finaly the refrigerator builds their character and we are done.

Oh, well, we were eaten up. My God! Still we made it, we penetrated inside. Now it's time to reactivate the enzymes.

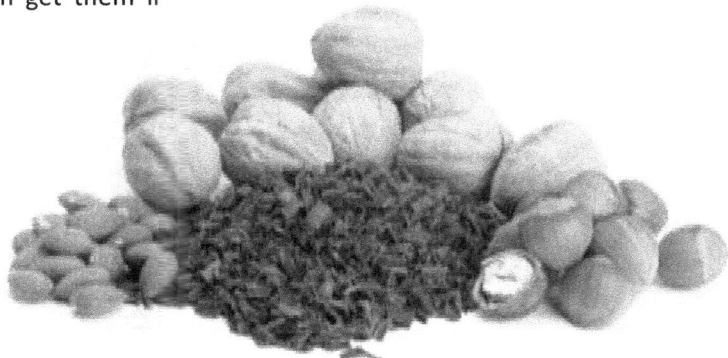

Dough for 4 pizzas:
500 g wholegrain Kamut flour,
yeast,
water salt

Mediterranea 1:
500 g ripe tomatoes,
1 pepper,
a bunch of asparaguses,
3-4 artichokes,
¼ kg champignons,
fresh basil and oregano,
unpasteurized olives and capres,
250 g cheese of raw milk
(goat' s and sheep's are the best)

Mediterranea 2:
instead of asparaguses,
artichokes and champignons,
eggplants,
zucchini and champignons, any fresh
vegetables: broccoli, cauliflower,
onion, leek...

PIZZA MEDITERRANA

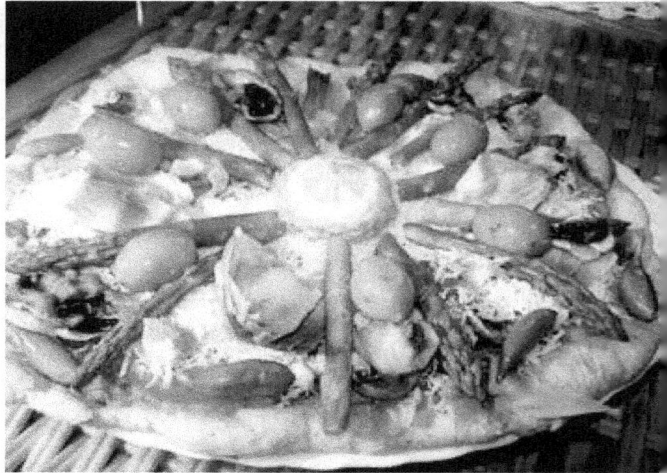

In pizzerias there are usually up to 100 and more different pizzas on the menu, but from a dietetic-medical point of view they are all the same – all consumed by fire. I will show you how to make the utmost healthy pizza, which has the most life in it. We will bake only the dough and certain vegetables, whereas the rest will remain fresh as was given to us by Mother Nature. You have never tried pizza like this in your life and when you learn the procedure, you will be delighted and make all the different pizzas you want...

Make the dough from Kamut flour, make 4 loaves, leave for at least

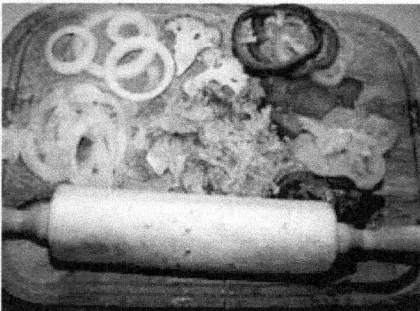

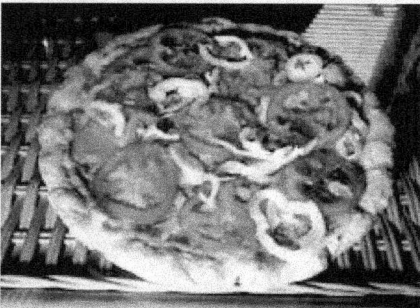

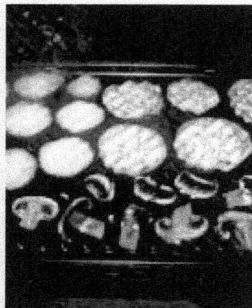

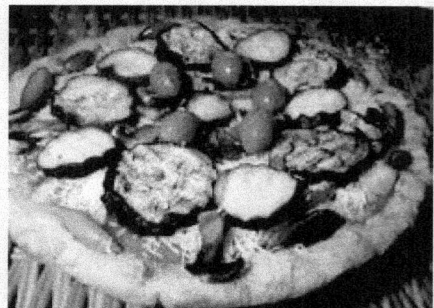

half an hour to rise and make round pizzas. Don't add oil to the dough and don't grease the baking tray – use Teflon tray. Now thinely slice zucchini, eggplants, mushrooms or other vegetable that needs heat to become edible and bake pizza at a relatively low temperature of 170ºC for a shorter period of time approx. 15 minutes, because we are baking dough only with some thinly sliced vegetables. Optionaly you can grill some vegetables (especially different mushrooms) and place them on pizza after dough is baked, this is how they do it in fine restaurants. Grill the vegetables without oil, use Teflon toaster grill. Anyway, at least one or two vegetables you should bake placed on top of the dough so the dough is soked and soft.

After our pizza is baked wait a minute or two to cool down a bit and spread any of tomato sauce from 4.th recipy. Now chop a bunch of fresh basil, oregano and a garlic clove, add virgin olive oil and spread delicious marinade over the pizza. Now lets prepare other vegetables. Make sure the tomatoes are ripe and soft – cut them into centimeter thick rings, soften them by partly squashing them and layer them on pizza. Slice up the peppers, onion, broccoli, cauliflower, leek or any similar vegetables into 3-4mm slices and roll them with a roller so that they soften and theres no need to bake them to taste well. Spread the vegetables over the most healthy pizza you ever had. **For the future there is a plan to put on the market a vegetable crusher with two rollers for softening vegetables. By simply turning the handle, the softening of stiffer vegetables will be made easier and smarter cooking will preserve numerous vitamins.**

What about cheese? Grate the cheese and sprinkle over the pizza. **If you prefer melted cheese you can serve it as a fondue.** You can also **sprinkle pizza with cheese and bake in an oven only from top** for 2-3 min at about 100°C, **only to melt the cheese**, but vigilantly watch through the window when cheese starts to melt and immediately take pizza out of the oven and serve it. On top of our super healthy pizza distribute olives and capers naturally conserved in saltwater. If you can't get them, demand them, and if you still don't get them stick the manufacturers' head in saltwater and hold for 60-90 seconds. Let them speak a few words, then repeat the procedure if necessary, they will learn. Just a joke!

Baby corn and peas are a specialty on a pizza. Fresh and young, they don't need cooking or steaming. They are steaming hot because of their youth. Baby peas and corn are picked earlier than usual, you have to capture the moment, when they mature, but aren't ripe yet, when they are full of sugars, sweet and delicious. Freeze some smaller packages for the winter, or end up on cans and at your funeral mass. Dear pizza lovers, we have managed to combine medicine with gourmet pleasures. Every day for a something new and at least 100 pizzas ahead of you...but the formula stays the same.

Spinach soup:
¾ kg potatoes or 300 g chickpeas,
300 g spinach,
½ celery root,
½ celery stalk,
parsley or parsnip,
½ onion or 2-3 shallots,
dill is a must,
1.5 dl sour cream,
parsley leaves,
garlic clove or chives,
cold pressed sunflower oil,
salt

Pumpkin soup:
1/2kg potatoes,
½ kg pumpkin,
2 yellow peppers,
1 onion,
celery root,
celery greens,
parsley with leaves,
1.5 dcl sour cream,
garlic clove,
sunflower oil,
salt,
spices

SPINACH AND PUMPKIN SOUP

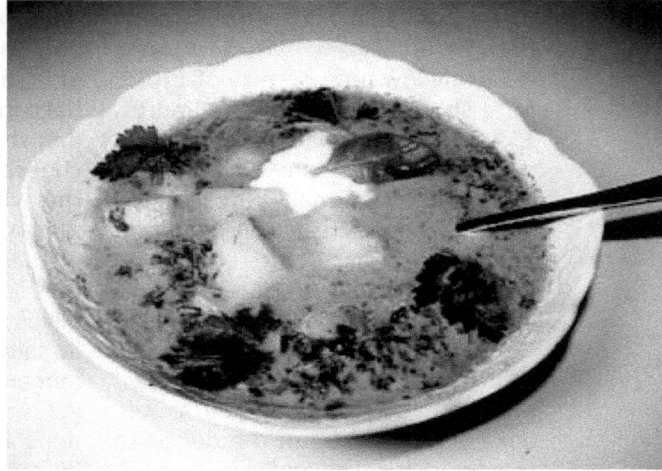

This is yet another popular soup which is prepared completely wrong according to most recipes. Today's gastronomy is like living in the 16th century; it competes for gold medals and makes specialties that turn into ashes. Why cook the vegetables, if they turn into poison by doing so? Dear cooks, why not question your old practice and change your mindset? Separate your greens into those, which need to go into the pot to become edible and those, which are edible as they are. Do you know the song 'Nothing Else Matters' by Metallica? Let's

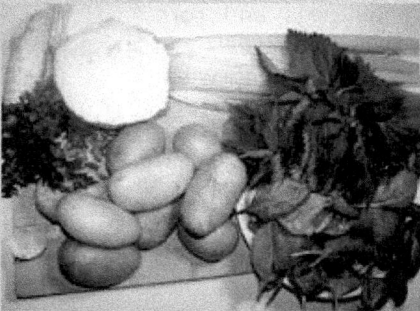

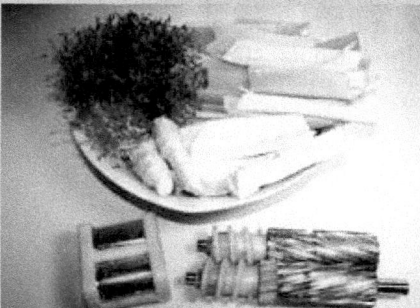

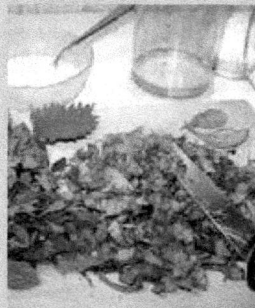

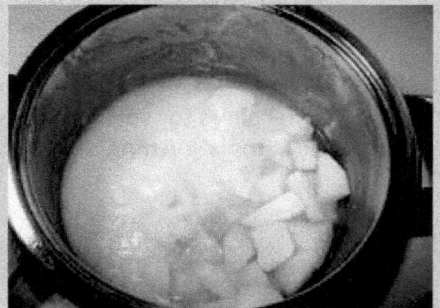

get on with the change.

Peel the potatoes, chop them up and cook in salted water. Leave them to cool a bit and blend one half of soup, leave the other half in cubes. That's our béchamel sauce. Chickpeas is great too, some even prefer it.

Sautee the onion. When the oil becomes motor oil, the sugars in the onion start to caramelize like making sugar for Coca-Cola and the healing effect of an onion is reduced like 1 divided by 10 in Maths. Add the spinach and slowly braise, so that the bountiful iron in spinach becomes old iron. Just don't eat the bicycles or old iron like some do.

And now for real: chop the spinach and blend it into purée. To make it easier, add some vegetable juice and sunflower oil. Chop the garlic, chives and parsley leaves and mix with the spinach. Here comes the face-off with which this soup will become healing – the highlight of pharmaceutical revelations. Use a juicer or mixer and a strainer. Squeeze the juice from the celery root and stalk, parsley and onion. Only a touch of onion, the key is celery. We know that celery soothes and calms the nerves, feeds the body and soul, parsley helps the mind and onion strengthens the heart and clears the veins. What else do you want? Ah, you want to eat.

Mix spinach and fresh juice with warm potato soup and add some spoons of sour cream. Don't forget the dill as it gives the final boost of flavour and serve soup at the right moment, when it is just temperature to serve, but the life in the vegetable juice is preserved, so it can continue to evolve into a higher life form.

Pumpkin soup you make in the same way: chop up the potatoes and pumpkin, cook them and partly squash. Juice the celery and parsley, chop up the peppers and onion, roll with a roller and add to the freshly squeezed juice.

Some like their soups hot. No problem. Here's a way of serving healing soups that most will enjoy. Serve separately cooked soup and freshly squeezed juice soup. First, pour in the bowl the hot soup, slowly sip it, which will make you warm, this is your starter. When the soup cools off a bit, pour into liquid medicine and in this way have it all...make it a gourmet ritual.

We have adequately divided the vegetables, cooked some, juiced, chopped or mixed the others. Why not use this dividing principle and make also other soups: pea, cabbage, onion, carrot, string beans, cauliflower, broccoli, etc...? Any hotchpotch of vegetables you can mix with healing juices, just let your imagination burst. Or make the stack raw and subsequently add: potatoes, noodles, stars, etc... Cooks, don't cook everything, be smart and be modern, become a new generation of conscious cooking artists. For inspiration here and there take a peep at the Medicine of Nature website, where you will find all sorts of good combinations and culinary innovations or just experiment on your own. Renaissance.

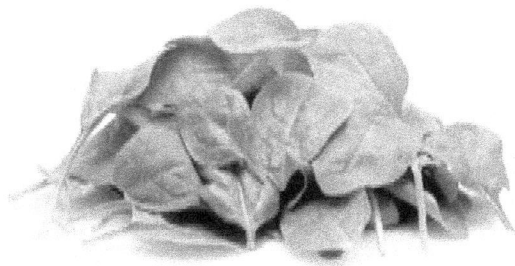

750 g tomato,
250 g colorful beans,
250 g seitan,
250 g Hokkaido pumpkin,
1 green pepper,
1 onion,
garlic clove,
50 g dry tomatoes,
3 tbs powdered red paprika,
1 tbs powdered onion,
soy sauce,
5-10 tbs sunflower oil,
2 bay leaves,
1 chili pepper,
ground cumin,
pepper,
grated sheep cheese if desired

RAINBOW CHILI

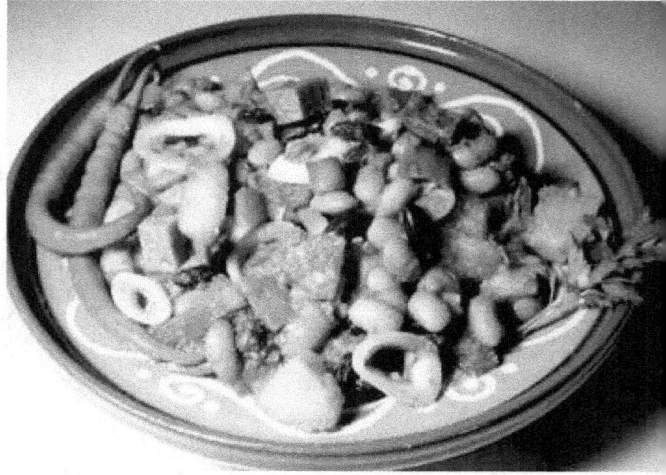

The colorful mixture of beans and vegetables on the plate remind us of a rainbow – the great heavenly flag. A rainbow is an international flag under which all living creatures on Earth travel through the universe. The divine force hangs it out in the rain as a sign of equality. The rain is sadness, the sun is joy and the rainbow a portal to the new era. Let the sun finally shine on all people and animals equally; this is the meaning behind the rainbow arch. Even animals are sad and experience joy, when we leave them at pastures, where they

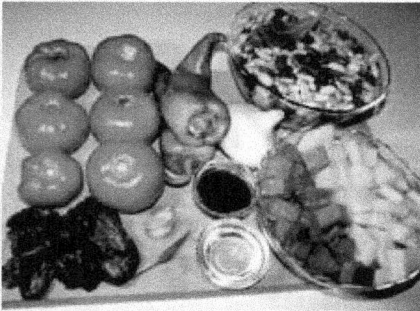

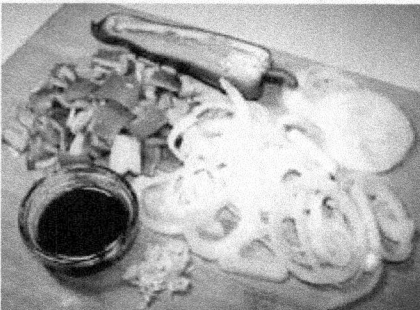

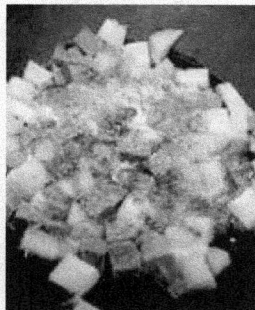

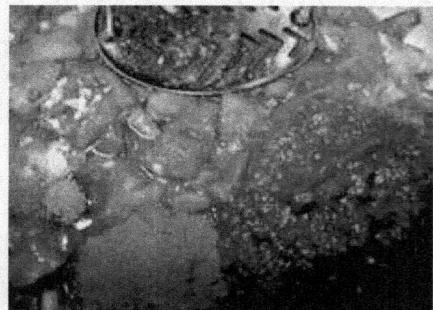

belong to enjoy another day. For the gift of milk for cheese we will thank them with due respect and rejoice in making a tasteful rainbow chili.

Bean mixture. Mix black, white, grey, red, colorful, any beans, possibly even chickpeas. Soak the mixture for 24 hours, even better let it sprout for two days. While soaking change water every now and then. Cook with two bay leaves, strain the water and let it cool of, before mixing in other ingredients.

Marinade. Cut the onion into rings and separate them with fingers, chop the peppers into centimeter cubes, finely chop the garlic. In a clay bowl pour over the three ingredients some table spoons of soy sauce and marinate at 50ºC for a half an hour in a drier or simpler: squash it with a roling pin.

Meat. Cube the seitan and Hokkaido pumpkin and braise for a little while on moderate fire without oil. Pour over the leftovers from the beans and season to taste. When choosing seitan, be picky and ask the seller which is recommended. Seitan is like meat, shallow without seasoning – use thousands of leaves mixture of spices. Instead of seitan, you can also use mushrooms with soy meat.

Cut the tomato into cubes and squash a bit. Use some clear tomato juice to soak the dry tomatoes and blend with a blender into sauce (you can add some cubes of raw Hokkaido pumpkin) and mix back in with the squashed tomato. Some spoons of powdered red paprika, a spoon of powdered onion, some chili, sunflower oil and the tomato sauce is 'ready'.

Mix in the bean mixture, marinated vegetables and stewed seitan with the tomato sauce, which binds everything together in a healthy, ethic dish. At the end season with pepper to your taste, add some cumin and serve. For the gourmets sprinkle some grated fresh cheese and enjoy your rainbow dish in peace. Make the flag flutter in the colors of the rainbow.

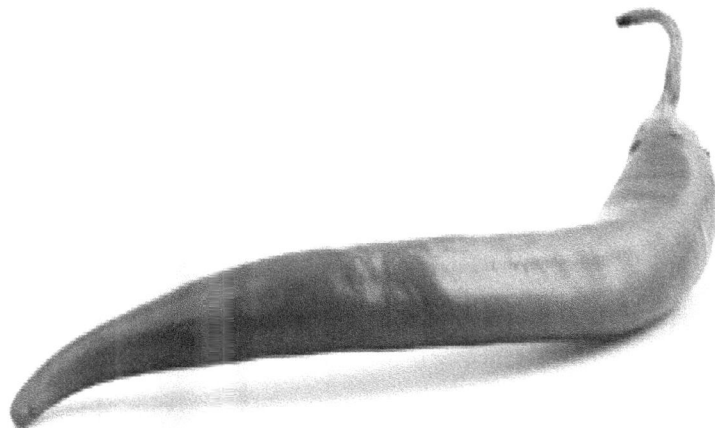

Moon chocolates:
100 g raw cocoa butter,
80 g coconut oil,
100 g honey = 3-4 tbs,
20 g powdered cocoa,
50 g hazelnuts,
50 g almonds,
50 g cocoa grains,
¼ ts powdered vanilla

Crunchy moon chocolates:
100 g raw cocoa butter,
80 g coconut oil,
100 g honey = 3-4 tbs,
20 g powdered cocoa,
crunchy mixture.
50 g sunflower seeds,
50 g hemp seeds,
50 g cocoa grains,
50 g chia seeds

5 star chocolates:
100 g cocoa butter,
40 g powdered cocoa,
7 tbs agave nectar,
200 g fresh cashews

MOON CHOCOLATES AND 5 STAR CHOCOLATES

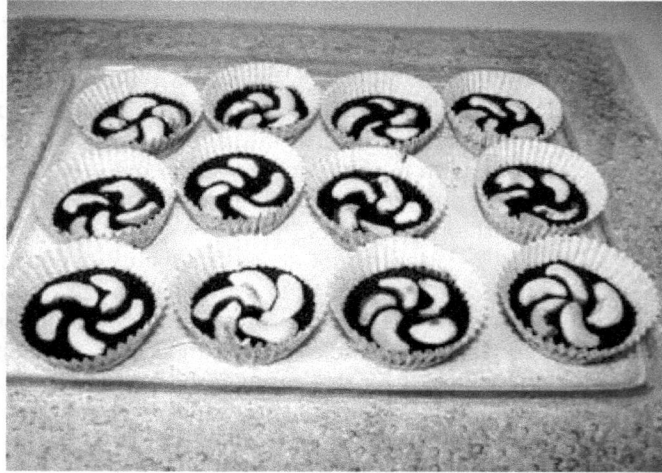

Moon lovers, chocolate lovers and all those in love, here comes a new passion. When you are moon walking or have love problems, don't jump through the window, walk to your refrigerator. You won't forget these nighttime strolls. Let passion carry you, even if you walk barefoot. (Make your own chocolates, even if you don't have the money for expensive ingredients.)

I discovered this recipe by chance, probably moon walking. Moon chocolates got their name from moon cycles. From a medical point of view, this is healthy fresh

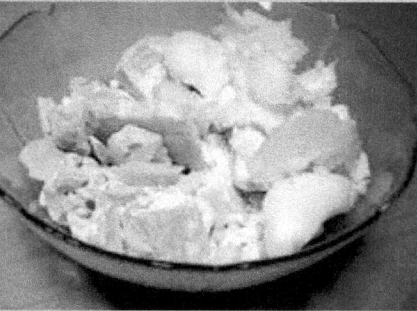

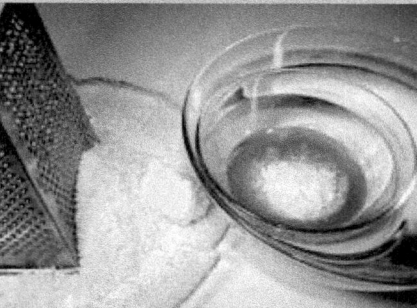

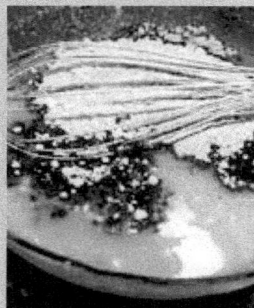

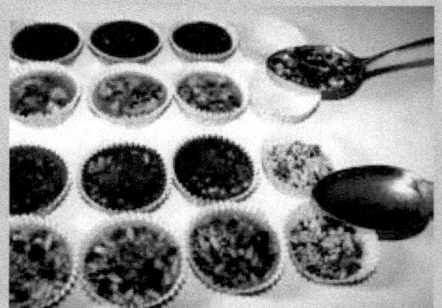

chocolate and belongs to the soft chocolate type. Ordinary chocolate contains cocoa butter with a melting point of 33ºC, whereas soft chocolate also contains cocoa butter with the melting point of 23ºC, which is why it melts even quicker in the mouth. It's like a smouldering French kiss. The key to good soft chocolate is the right ratio between the both, 100:80. If there is too much coconut oil, the chocolate kiss is too greasy, if you overdo the cocoa butter it will be coarse – so do the weighing.

First grate the cocoa butter and whisk it in a double bowl until melted. Make sure that the water does not enter the dish. Make the water rather warm in the lower bowl, but not hot, to ensure that the butter remains virgin fresh. Rather change the water several times than melt over boiled water. When the cocoa butter is melted, add the coconut oil, which becomes liquid already at room temperature. Or you can also use the drier for the melting of butter, simply set the temperature at 42ºC.

Grind half the hazelnuts and almonds, chop up the other half – with short impulses in the food processor. Mix honey, vanilla, ground, chopped hazelnuts and almonds, cocoa grains in the melted butter and whisk. Split the batter into two even parts, one made up of light chocolate and in the other part mix in the powdered cocoa to get dark chocolate. Pour the chocolates into mignon papers, place in the refrigeratorand after 10 minutes, when it starts to harden, sink a whole almond on top, hazelnut and sprinkle over cocoa grains. Occasionally different comets will fly into chocolates: Pecans, pistachios, raw cashews, macadamia nuts, pine nuts, coconut...

Crunchy moon chocolates change our memories forever. A mixture of equal parts of sunflower seeds, hemp seeds, cocoa grains and chia is the recipe for crunchy chocolates. Fill up the mignon papers with a mixture of seeds and pour over soft chocolate. Keep the chocolates in the refrigerator for at least 2 hours, before you begin moon walking. The taste is simple heavenly!

5 star chocolates were brought to Earth by the astronauts from the last Apollo mission. The star made of cashews soaked in chocolate was found on a low bush similar to a Christmas star. Thank God the fresh cashews from the moon have sprouted and we can pick the tasteful fruit today. If we fold the cashews next to each other we get the most beautiful five-armed star. First pour in the chocolate and then fold the stars. Make dark chocolate and pour 2 teaspoons in each mignon paper, leave for a couple of minutes to thicken and make the stars. When the astronauts left the moon, they spotted a cow in the distance through the window of their spaceship. It was grazing on one of the moon hills. It was dark purple. They waved at it, but it didn't comprehend the meaning of goodbye.

Do you know why people don't travel to the moon anymore? Because the way to the refrigerator, where there is a tray of moon chocolates and tasteful stars is so much closer. Full moon and honey moon is approaching. The astronauts agree, nod their heads, slowly take off their space suits and with great pleasure unwrap the chocolates from their mignon papers.

Strawberry parfait:
1/2 kg strawberry,
½ bananas,
1 mango,
2 dl sweet cream
(vegans can use coconut oil),
powdered vanilla,
cocoa beans

Fairy-tale parfait:
cup of blueberries,
honey,
homemade kefir,
cup of raspberries,
wood strawberry,
ome apricots,
sour cream,
agave nectar

Parfait from berries are colorful:
blueberries,
raspberries,
wood strawberries,
currant,
gooseberry,
a lot of honey;
vanilla cream
according to recipe no. 14,
fresh chocolate...

SPRING PARFAIT

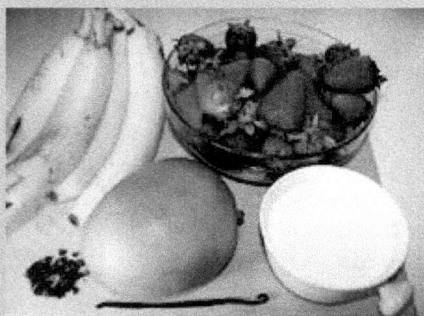

Imagine a typical morning deep in the jungle with the sun ray penetrating through the leaves. Two chimpanzees Mary and Jo are munching on a bunch of bananas high in the palm treetops. I-i-i-i-i-i, i-i-i-i- Mary found a mango, u-u-u-u-u-u-a-a-a-a-a Jo revealed her perfect white teeth with a smile with mango in one hand and a juicy papaya in the other. AaaAAAAAAAAAAAaaaaaaaaa Who goes there? Tarzan, of course...

arfait comes from French and means perfect, the perfect fruit cream, perfect breakfast, perfect snack, perfect

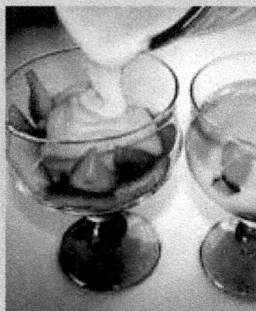

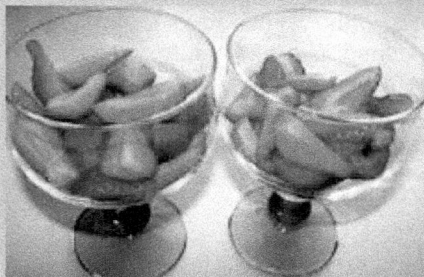

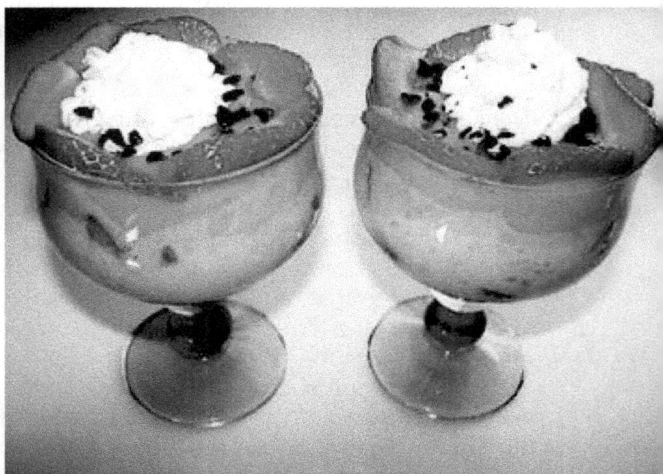

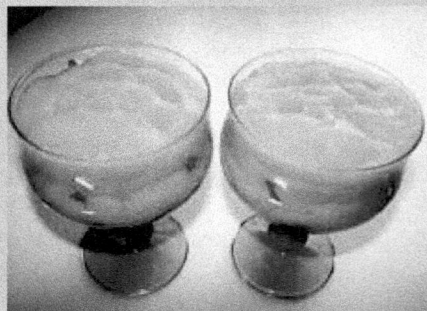

lunch. Parfait also looks perfect: colorful layers of fruit cream with fruit bits in tall glasses with cream and chocolate on top.

Mix some strawberries in the mixer, cup some up to quarters, rings or slices, whatever you desire in the fresh morning. Pour the strawberry cream into the glasses and dip the strawberry pieces in the cream. Than blend the bananas, sweet cream, powdered vanilla and pour in the second layer. Dip some banana rings in the cream. To make the cream extra saucy, you can whisk the cream a little beforehand. Mix in the mango, pour in the third layer, some whipped cream on top, cocoa beans and almond leaves – mamma mia! It is not enough for your breakfast you will say? Serve it with a few croissants filled with natural marmelade...

We can make similar fairy-tale creams out of berries. Let's try next recipe: make the first layer out of blueberries and honey, pour in the fairy-tale glass and sprinkle over some whole blueberries. Don't put off a layer of homemade kefir or yogurt, as blueberries simply love it. Raspberries are getting ready to jump into the glass. It's rather tall, some land and get squashed, others land safely and intact. Also partially blend a layer of wood strawberries, leave some intact and allow 3 halves of apricots to float on top loaded with sour cream. Seal off the fairy-tale parfait with a topped spoon of agave nectar.

The fresh mornings in the embrace of a forest are the most beautiful. If we have time, we can take a walk to load up on some oxygen, perhaps meet someone famous. E-e-e-e-e-e-e-e-e, gre-e-e-e-e-e-ens, gre-e-e-e-e-ens...Who goes there? Mrs. Bouthenko is climbing! Of course – balm leaf or mint for decoration. Aaaaa-AAAAAAAAAA-aaaaaaaaaaa

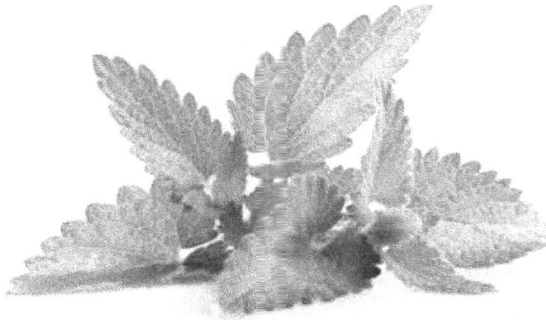

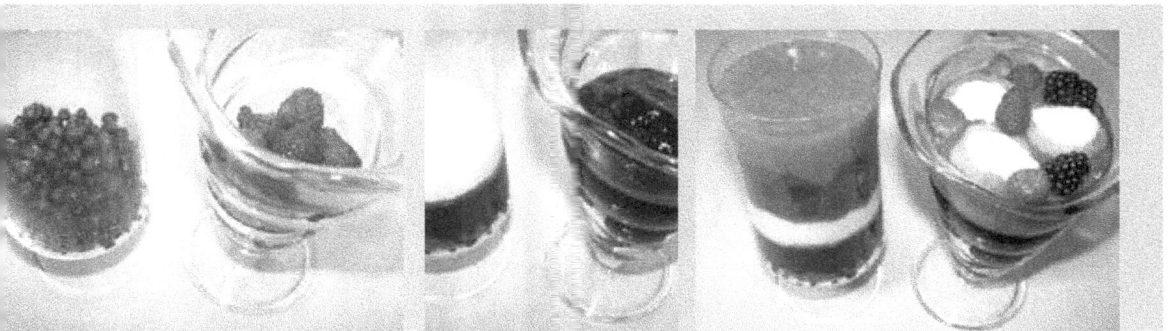

Dandelion salad:
a larg bowl of dandelion,
a medium bowl of rampion,
a smaller bowl of rocket,
3-4 potatoes,
1 avocado,
a bowl of dandelion flowers,
cold pressed sunflower oil,
vinegar,
lemon juice,
salt

Parsley salad:
400 g young parsley leaves,
100 g of young celery leaves and or
French parsley,
100 g alfalfa sprouts,
300 g beans,
50 g rocket,
2 onions,
cold pressed pumpkin or virgin olive
oil,
vinegar,
lemon juice,
salt,
pepper

DANDELION AND PARSLEY SALAD

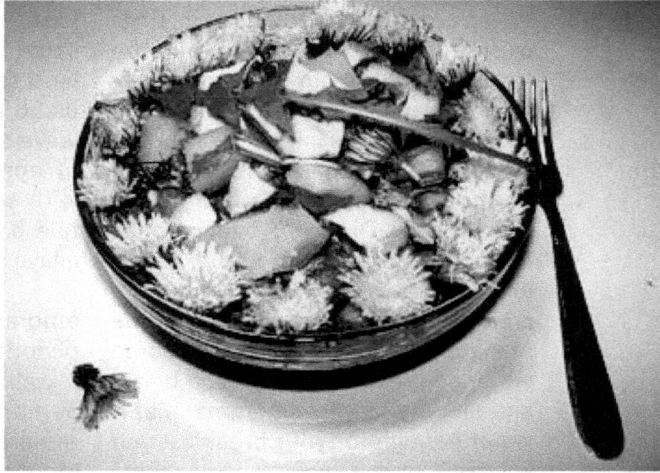

A little joke in the previous recipe. Mrs. Victoria Bouthenko is an independent researcher and scientist, who warns the Western world about the deficit of greens in our nutrition. Chimpanzees eat a lot of buds and green leaves, around 40%. The modern human being should, according to my estimates, consume around 20% of greens and buds. Green-leaved vegetables are very tasty, if they are ecologically-grown and well combined, prepared with feeling.

Dandelion is no. 1 among the self-grown, wild food. It grows in abundance,

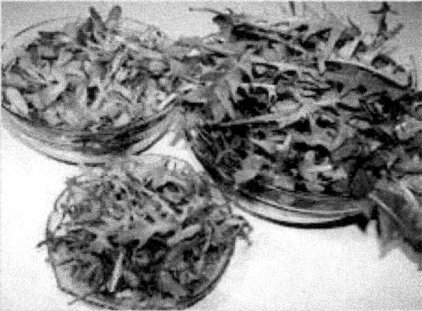

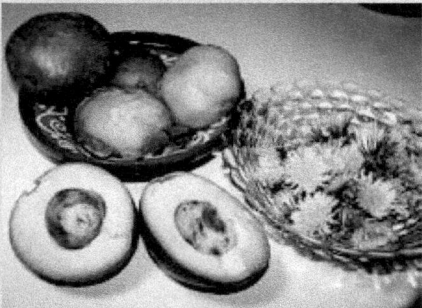

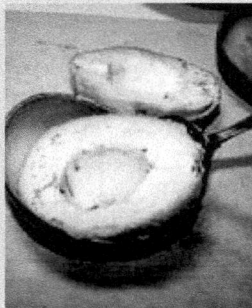

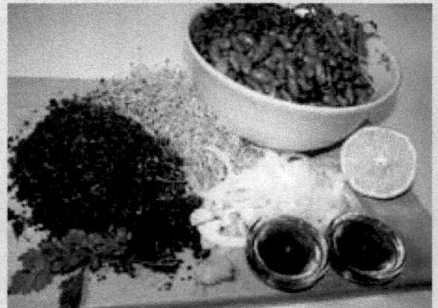

it is tasty, healing and, if combined in a bowl with rampion and rocket, the salad is perfect. **Dandelion is a little stringy, but with soft rampion, it becomes the best pair.** Mrs. Bouthenko is nodding her head. I have tried a great deal of dandelion salads, I have mixed all sorts of greens, but I tell you that the following recipe is by far the best.

Cut up the potatoes and cook. Rinse our green-leaved trio, cut up and stir. Make sure the avocado is ripe, best is buttery one. Cut it in half, remove the stone and spoon out the flesh in thin leaves. Now let's add some dandelion blossoms, which we don't rinse in water, but only blow during picking. **When I tried dandelion blossoms for the first time, I couldn't believe the taste and ever since I haven't eaten a salad without dandelion blossoms.** Eating dandelion blossoms instead of eggs is incomparably healthier. A blossom is the carrier of a new plant, how wouldn't it be healthy? Add oil, lemon, vinegar, salt and stir well for the avocado to butter the salad. Decorate the edge of the bowl with yellow dandelion blossoms. Bon appétit!

In the next salad parsley is not a spice, but the main ingredient. It's not a bean salad with parsley, but parsley salad with beans. The ratio is reversed and the flavor with careful preparation far better than the classic version. Organically grown parsley has that sweet savory bitterness to it compared to the artificially grown, which simply tastes bitter. Chew up a branch, when you buy it. If you can't find good homemade parsley, you can grow it yourself in a pot. There's another mystery, which is to make sure that the parsley leaves are young and juicy. The exceptional taste of this salad comes from the young celery leaves, which look a lot like parsley. This is another super food. If you can't get young celery leaves in supermarkets, it's best if you grow it yourself, because if you will use old celery leaves which are usually on market, you won't be as passionate about this salad as I am.

Cook the beans with bay leaves, cool off and mix with chopped parsley and young celery leaves. **Finely chop the parsley to release the juice, which is the healing ingredient, the very heart of the salad.** Really try chopping up the parsley, because it will be easier to chew and the salad will taste better. Cut the onion into rings and separate them with fingers. Add alfalfa sprouts, lemon juice, vinegar, oil and salt. The cold pressed pumpkin oil was pressed with love just for this aromatic salad. **With these two recipes we have come closer to our ancient lives in the jungle.** Bon appétit!

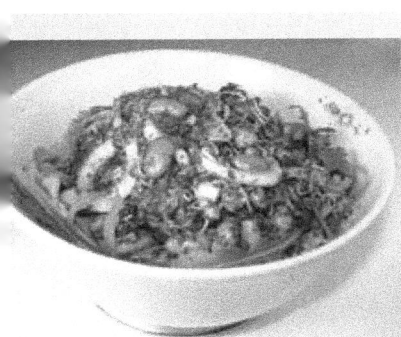

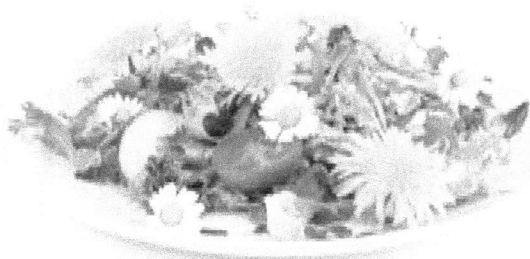

Seafood pizza:
1 small zucchini,
3 ripe tomatoes,
50 g dry tomatoes,
1 pepper,
some cauliflower,
3-4 artichokes,
200 g tofu,
200 g fresh cheese,
20 g wakame algae,
20 dulse algae,
olives,
capers,
fresh basil,
oregano,
virgin olive oil

Pizza vegetariana:
3 ripe tomatoes,
100 g cherry tomatoes,
50 g dry tomatoes,
1 pepper,
1 onion,
200 g goat or sheep cheese,
200 g seitan,
baby peas and corn,
cauliflower,
broccoli,
aladdin,
olives,
bunch of basil,
garlic clove,
olive oil

Spinach – 4 cheeses
200 g spinach,
3 tbs sour cream,
4 different fresh cheeses – ripened
and fresh,
cauliflower,
broccoli,
aladdin,
baby corn,
bunch of parsley
leaves,
rocket, garlic,
soy sauce,
sunflower oil
(don't use all the ingredients,
these are only ideas for the finest
combinations.)

SEAFOOD PIZZA, VEGETARIANA, SPINACH AND 4 CHEESES

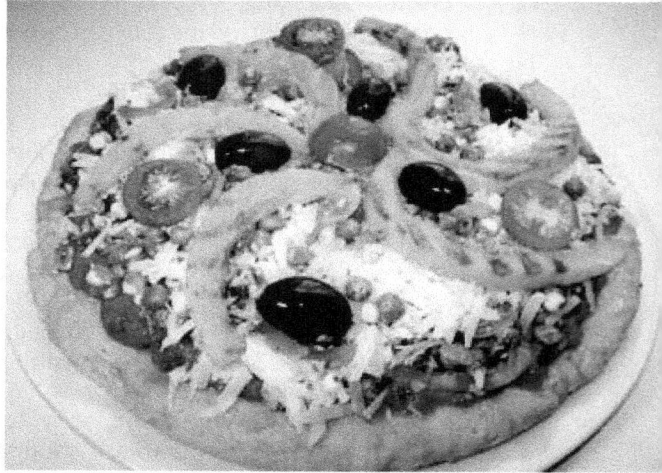

The pizza world is huge, a small culinary solar system with countless planets. We will describe some of the most popular pizzas, which can satisfy the most, let's say 90% of the Earth's inhabitants. You can make any pizza for your loved ones. For those who like their meat, make it vegetarian. If you are hosting aliens, serve them with spinach. When you are wooing, get some shrimps ready for the seafood version.

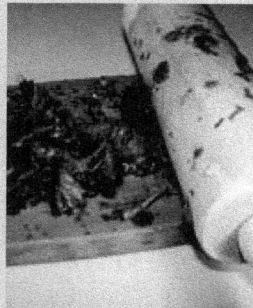

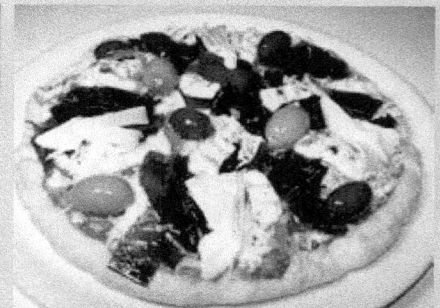

Cut the tofu into centimeter slices, then to crescents)))))). Grill the shrimps for 5 minutes in a toaster so that they get ribs from the grill. Let them rest in a marinade of soaked algs and seasoning. If well-seasoned, they should taste like genuine white meat, so spread them over the pizza with soaked algae. **Algae give the pizza a genuine taste of the sea, because the oceans are flowing through algae.**

Cut the tomatoes into rings and squash them so that they release their juice. Pressure works on tomatoes similarly as temperature, it allows the juice to come, but preserves the vitamins. In a blender the purée would jellify, because tomatoes contain pectin. Use the juice to soak the dry tomatoes, then blend it into a sauce with a blender, add the pieces of squashed tomatoes, chopped basil, oregano, virgin olive oil, garlic and salt. Dry tomatoes thicken the sauce, there are fresh herbs... mmmmh, that smells good! **A genuine sauce – "Salsa vera"**

'Put together' the seafood pizza following recipe 16. Baked Kamut dough baked with sliced zucchini, fresh salsa, marinated sliced pepper and cauliflower, revived algae, grated cheese, grilled shrimp, unpasteurized olives, capers...

Vegetariana: Marinate the vegetables in a couple of spoons of soy sauce: thinly grated pepper, cauliflower, broccoli, aladdin, onion rings, sweet peas, baby corn and ripe cherry tomatoes. At 42ºC the vegetables soften, but retain the right amount of crunchiness. If we put seitan on a vegetariana, it becomes classic pizza. It has no correlation with Satan, quite the contrary, it replaces red meat. Cut it a little thicker than ham and roast in its juice. It becomes a little more homely, if we grill vegetarian sausages without oil. You can get them in any health food store.

Spinach and 4 cheeses: Distribute the spinach sauce (recipe 3) on the dough, add chopped parsley, rocket and fresh herbs according to your taste. Marinate some spinach leaves together with cauliflower. Aladdin, corn... Distribute the cheese slices, white cheese cubes, bits of cheese sauce like in recipe no. 8.

Mexicana is pizza with beans – you know ketchup and ajvar. Devil's pizza likes Tabasco and chili... I think I have given you enough information on the world of healthy pizzas, you are in the space rocket yourself, so find your own planet.

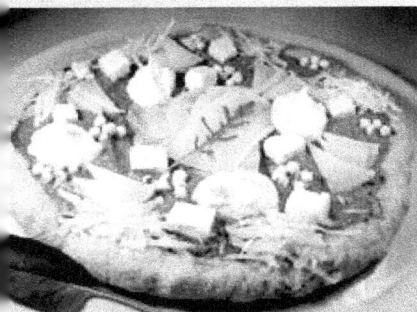

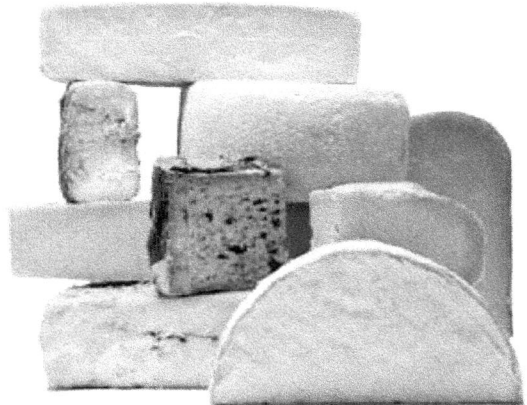

Chickpea hummus:
500 g chickpeas,
some bay leaves,
250 g carrots,
5-8 tbs tahini
paste from sprouted sesame,
parsley root and leaves,
1 dl virgin olive oil,
juice of 1 lemon,
2 garlic cloves,
some spoons of soy sauce,
1 ts powdered red pepper,
ground cumin,
ground pepper,
fist of pine nuts

Pea puree:
300 g dry peas,
smaller celery stalk
or half of a large one,
1 ripe avocado,
2-3 mint branches,
cold pressed sunflower oil,
salt,
pepper,
extras:
asparagus with raw butter, green
lettuce leaves,
rocket...

VITAMIN ENRICHED HUMMUS AND PEA PUREE

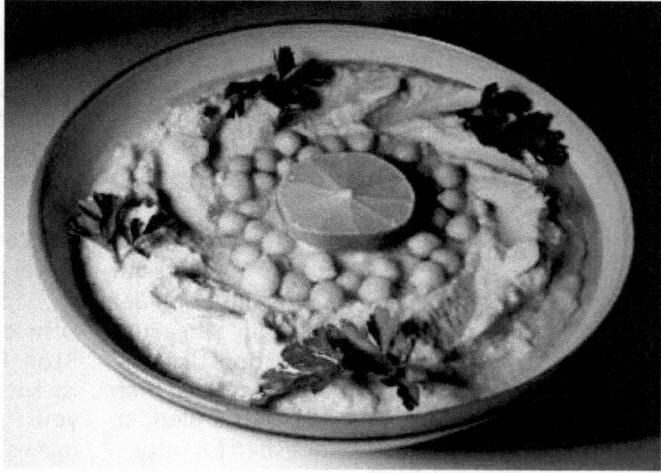

The home of hummus is the Near East, Arabian Peninsula, Israel, Palestine, Lybia, Syria, Jordan... Spirally served chickpea dish is so popular over there that there are many restaurants specialized only in hummus. The doctor has carefully examined chickpeas and determined that it is missing carrots. Pea puree is one of the best doctor's prescriptions. Both recipes are an excellent way how to instill life in puree: vitamins, minerals and enzymes.

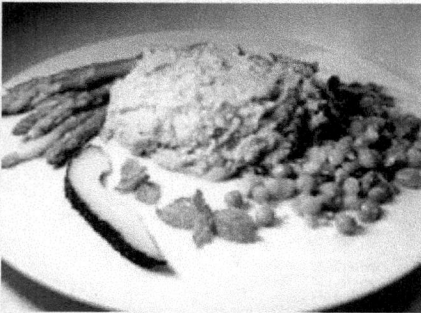

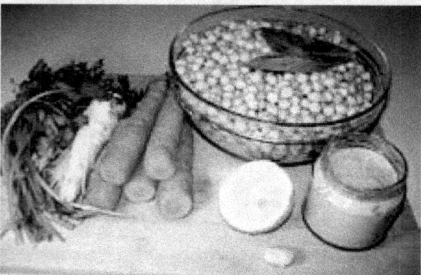

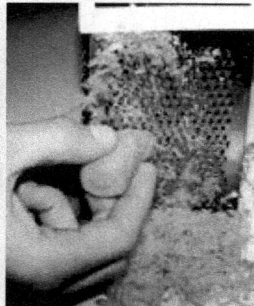

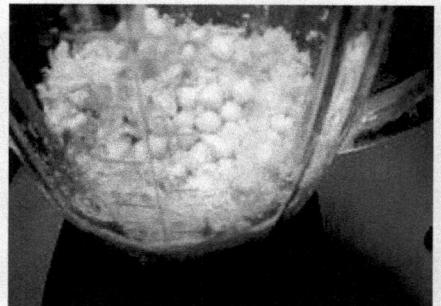

We will begin the recipe with a smaller improvement – tahini paste from sprouted sesame. Usually sesame is fried, we on the other hand are going to sprout it for 2-3 days, then mix with oil and salt in a blender. **Don't destroy food, learn to glorify the life in it regardless of the tradition.** Soak the chickpeas for 12-24 hours and cook with bay leaves. In a powerful blender first blend the carrots, parsley root, lemon juice, soy sauce, olive oil and a ladle of chickpea soup. Slowly add the warm chickpeas, sprouted tahini, ground cumin, spices and blend into paste. Serve as shown on the picture with the olive oil in the middle and a handful of chickpea grain. Adorn with parsley and sprinkle over pine nuts. If you leave the hummus overnight in the refrigerator it is even better the next day. If we don't like the texture, we can make traditional hummus with fresh tahini paste and nibble on some vegetables with it. Bil-hene-il-ošife! Enjoy! Two camels are already on the horizon...

We follow the same procedure to make pea puree: soak the dry peas overnight, cook, cool off a bit and blehind with celery stalk, avocado, sunflower oil, spices and the other ingredients. **Pea puree made this way is delicious and could be as popular as Hummus.** Serve the puree with cooked asparagus, whole pea beans and raw butter. Mix the raw and cooked at just the right time so that the final temperature when serving the dish is a little above body temperature. Revolution on your plates. Spread the word about vitamin-enriched purees around the world.

Since we are speaking of peas, here is yet another recipe. **Summer pea soup is 100% raw, easy to make and very good. You don't need to cook baby peas, if you pick it early, when it is still full of sugars.** The peas are a little smaller, but richer... you know what I mean. Pluck some cucumbers in the garden, colorful peppers and celery stalk. Blend and sift. Cube the avocado and blend into creamy soup. Squash some tomatoes, add salt, some table spoons of olive oil, parsley leaves, cup of baby peas and the summer pea soup for the late afternoon refreshment is on the garden table.

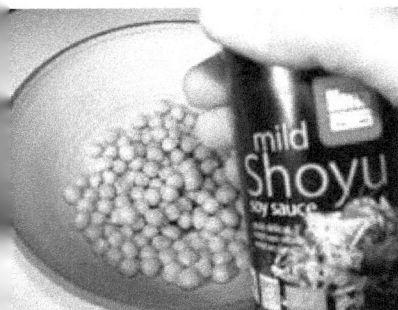

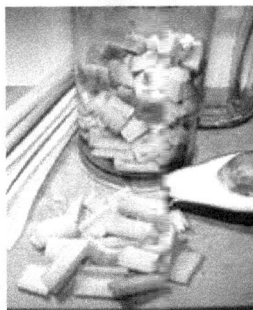

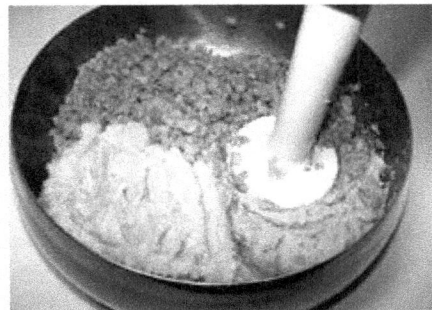

Stuffed peppers:
12 larger peppers,
50 g buckwheat =
100 g buckwheat sprouts,
50 g amaranth =
100 g amaranth sprouts,
100 g ripened cheese,
250 g mushrooms,
100 g soy meat,
2 tomatoes,
60-70 g dry tomatoes,
1 onion,
1 zucchini,
garlic,
parsley leaves,
7-9 tbs olive oil,
2 ts powdered red paprika,
coriander,
marjoram,
thyme,
pepper,
oy sauce

Stuffed tomatoes:
8 larger ripe tomatoes,
50 g dry tomato,
100 g buckwheat =
200 g buckwheat sprouts,
100 g ground walnuts,
a slice of Hokkaido pumpkin,
smaller onion,
parsley leaves,
20 g arame algae,
olive or walnut oil,
salt

STUFFED PEPPERS AND TOMATOES

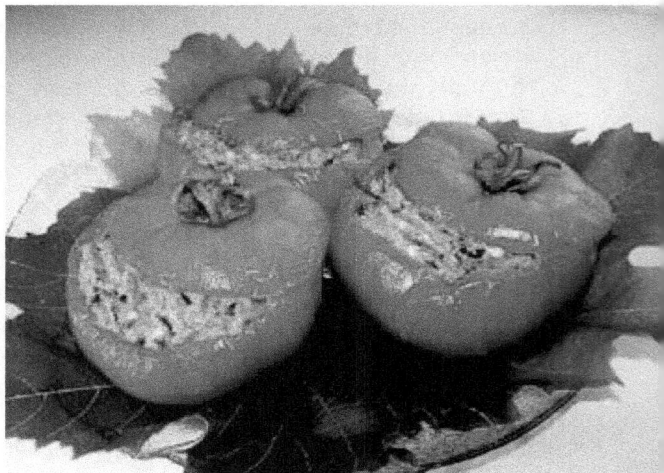

India, the Near East, Mediterranean, Australia, America, Scandinavia; the whole world has heard of stuffed peppers, but not like this. I haven't found a truly healthy recipe for stuffed tomatoes no matter what the name of the recipe promises! I've checked over hundreds of recipes and it's all the same; baking, cooking, braising, cooking and destroying all that's good in this paradise fruit. Our peppers and tomatoes are soft, tasty and juicy. The only thing braised are the mushrooms and soy meat in the peppers whereas

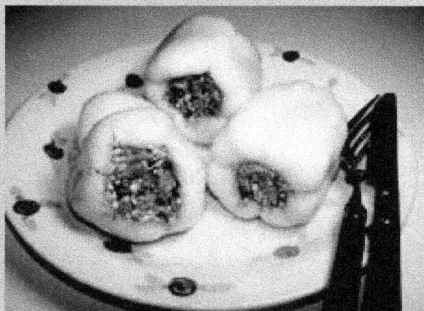
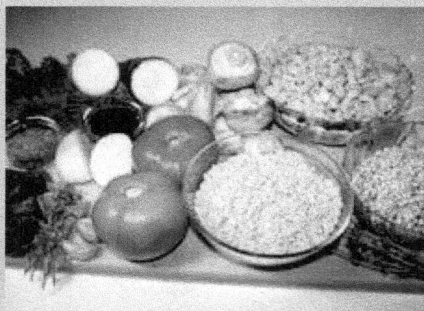
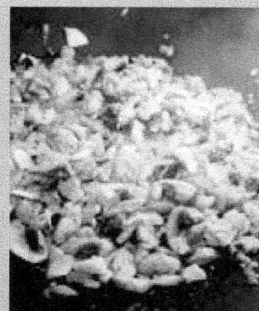

the tomatoes remain 100% raw and full of vitamins. **How do we achieve this? The key is the recipe, of course. We use really ripe tomatoes, which are finally softened by moderate heat in a drier. At the temperature of 47ºC in 8 hours the tomatoes soften up like they have been just removed from the oven.** Instead of high temperature and short time of cooking we use lower temperature and more time. **The peppers are somewhat more complicated, so we treat them with ice crystals in a freezer, which soften the peppers similarly as baking would.** After a brief freeze (1-2 hours) we stuff the peppers and heat them in a food drier. The final effect is identical, juicy stuffed peppers – you' be surprised. This recipe is worth a million dollars.

First, here is the recipe for stuffed peppers. Remove the stems and seeds from the peppers and soften them in a freezer for an hour or so. With this short-term freezing we preserve 80% of the vitamins compared to baking which doesn't preserve even 1%. There is a belief that a part of vitamin C is preserved at high temperatures, according to some positive tests, but there is no life in that vitamin – the laboratory vitamin tests are invalid.

Stuff the peppers with a mixture of sprouts, mushrooms, soy, fresh vegetables and spices. Soak the soy meat for a couple of minutes and dry in a wok with champignons, shitake, boletus or chanterelles. Make the tomato sauce in the same way as for a pizza. We have sprouted the buckwheat and amaranth for 48 hours, you can also sprout quinoa. Finely chop the garlic, onion and parsley leaves, grate the fresh zucchini and cheese and mix all the ingredients, season, pepper, etc. When the peppers are frozen, remove them from the freezer, stuff, heat in a drier to an appropriate temperature and serve. We can also stuff the peppers with a mixture of rise and fresh vegetables or mashed legumes and fresh vegetables. Experiment!

My favorites are stuffed tomatoes. Artificial tomatoes are unlikely to soften, they are normally stiff as if they had gone through plastic surgery – throw them away and grow your own in the garden. Cut the tomatoes under the stem, spoon out the tomato meat, and soften in a drier for 8 hours (don't forget the lids). Chop up the tomato flesh and strain with a strainer. Clear tomato juice is very healthy, so make it your appetizer – bottoms up! Divide the stuffing into two parts. Blend with a blender half of the removed tomato flesh, half of sprouted buckwheat, dry tomato and a slice of Hokkaido pumpkin. Chop up the other half of walnuts together with the onion and

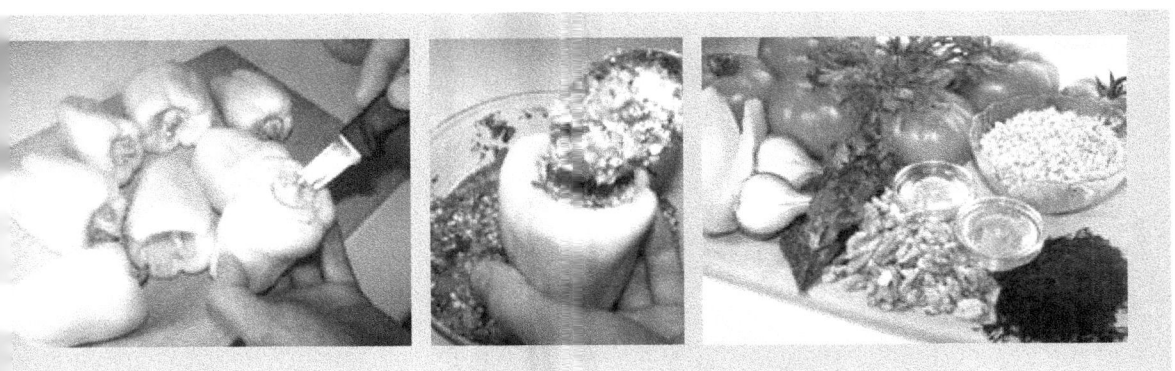

56

parsley leaves. Add the remaining half of buckwheat sprouts, ground arame algae, oil, spices and mix all the ingredients. While the tomatoes are 'baking', leave the stuffing at room temperature for the flavors to soak in. After eight hours stuff the tomatoes, heat in a drier for 20 minutes and serve. Stuffed tomatoes are incredible.

Let's get organized, we won't spend any more time than with normal recipes, in fact we'll live some 20 years longer. Do you know how many people on your continent succumb to cancer each year? Millions! **Let's be wise and book the ticket to paradise in advance. This recipe is worth a million dollars.**

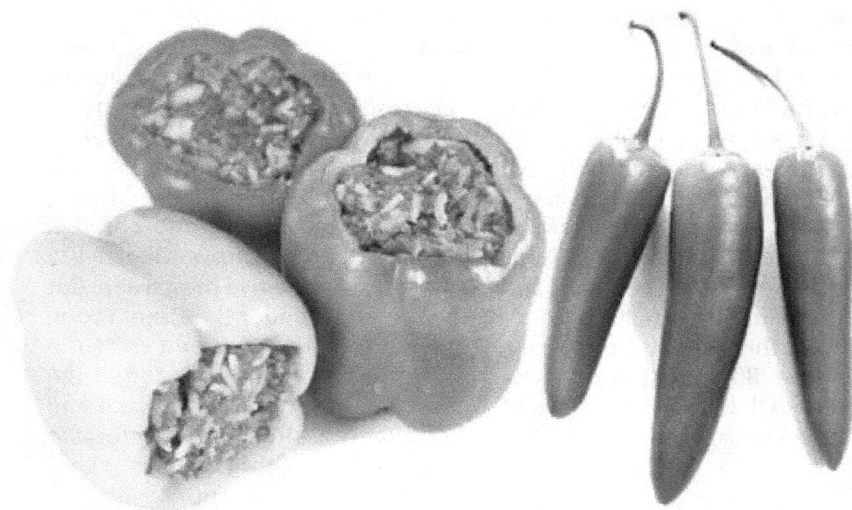

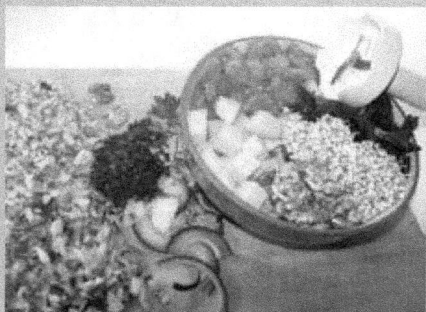

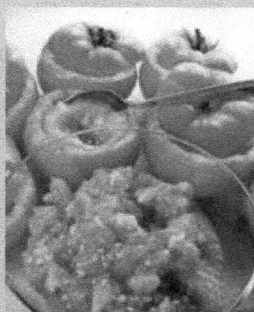

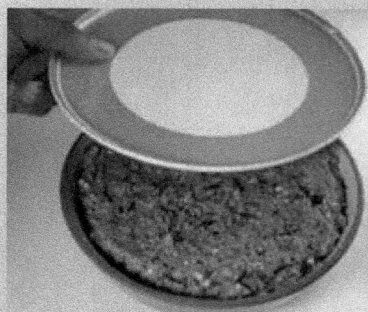

Dough for the rolls:
make the wholesome or pastry dough at home or buy it, but request the complaint's book in which you can clearly request wholesome dough without conservatives. You will get it, if you persevere. Salt.

Apple strudel:
4 larger apples of sweet-sour sort, 100 -150g ground hazelnuts, 100g raisins, a couple of spoons of honey, cinnamon, cloves, vanilla, perhaps a pear instead of an apple to sweeten the strudel

Poppy strudel:
500g ground poppy, 100g walnuts or pecans, 2 bananas, 5 tbs coconut oil, 100g date nuts or 5 tbs honey, vanilla

Cheese strudel:
500g fresh unprocessed white cottage cheese, 1dcl natural sweet cream, 100g raisins, vanilla, grated ecological orange peel

Walnut strudel:
300g walnuts, 200g pecans, 1dcl sweet cream, 4-5 tbs honey, ½ ts cinnamon, pinch of nutmeg, vanilla clove, grated ecological lemon peel, 100g sultana raisins or fresh chocolate

APPLE, POPPY, WALNUT AND CHEESE STRUDEL

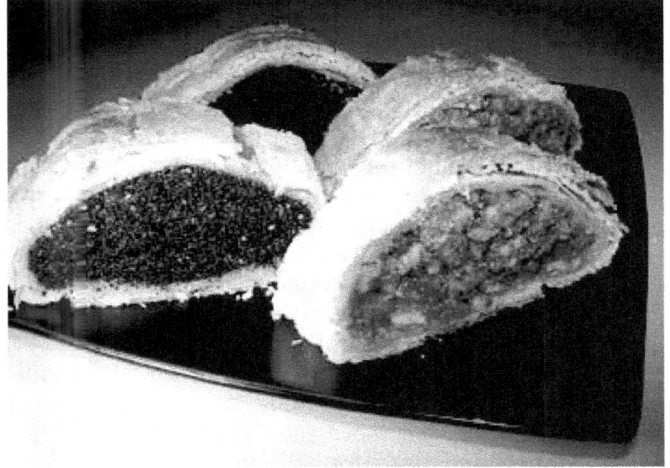

This is one of the most representative recipes in the book, especially for bakers. It best depicts the combination of classical baking and healthy raw food. For a lot of people baking desserts and cakes is a passionate hobby For them, this recipe gives them a chance to greatly enrich their hobby and to put their health at the number one priority. When people heard of preparing strudels in this way, they immediately wanted to purchase the recipe book, which was at the time still being written.

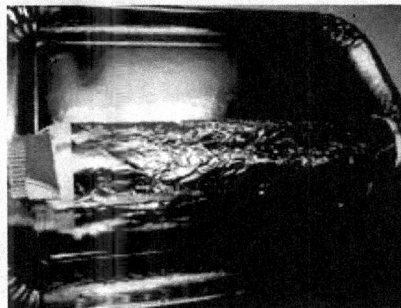

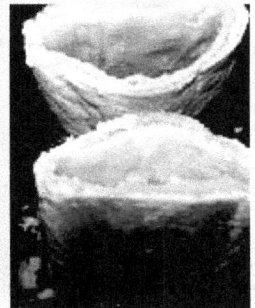

Once they tried them, they all said that from then on they would only make various strudels in this way. Without further ado, let's get to it.

We will roll the dough into a tube and bake it without the filling. We will add the fresh prepared filling later and in this way preserve the life and the rich flavor of natural ingredients. If we wish to bake the dough in the shape of a tube, we need something to keep the form. **Roll a small kitchen cloth or 2-3 kitchen towels and wrap it in tin foil.** Now wrap this strange roll into the dough as if it was the filling. The number of cloths depends on the amount of filling we wish to have in the dough. Dry the dough in the oven at 150°C for some 15 min, remove from the oven, carefully remove the cloths, but leave the foil in the dough and bake for additional 10-15 minutes at 180°C, depending on the oven. **We left the foil inside to imitate the filling so that the dough does not turn brown inside and remains soft.** This strudel will bake faster than ordinary strudel, because it has no filling and the end product is identical – crust on the outside and light yellow colour on the inside. Once it bakes, cut it in half in the middle and fill.

While the dough is baking, we prepare one of the fillings for the strudel. For apple strudel peel the apples, grate about a half finely, half coarse, add the raisins, cinnamon, honey and other spices. Don't soak the raisins, they will happily soak up the juice from the apples and do us a favour. The filling is done in a matter of minutes. You can also use the apples from the natural compote.

For poppy strudel blend the walnuts, bananas, coconut oil and spices and only then add the ground poppy seeds and mix with a spoon so that the poppy does not become bitter. It's best to prepare the filling ahead of time, so it can stand for a while or place the strudel in the refrigerator for a couple of hours before serving it.

The fantastic cheese strudel is made of homemade cottage cheese and sweet cream. The filling is made before the dough is baked, just mix all the ingredients in a bowl and that's it.

Grind most of the walnuts for the walnut strudel, chop up a few, you can also mix in some pieces of fresh chocolate or sultana raisins. **Walnuts and pecans are an exceptionally good company – friends forewer.** Spices and aromas are also important, they give that final twist. Mix them precisely with taste: grate a little lemon peel, pinch of nutmeg, some rum, vanilla, anything... **You can prepare the filling the way you**

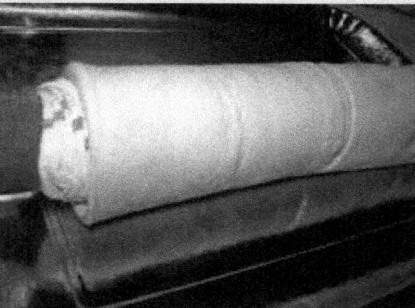

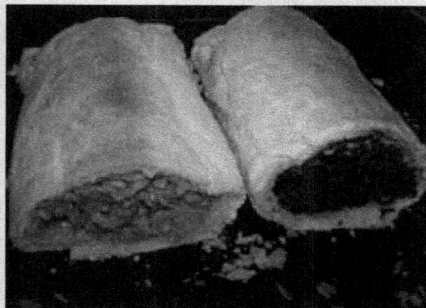

make it normally, it is the baking procedure, which is innovative.

The quality of the walnuts is extremely important. Inside husked walnuts, which stand on market shelves for months the fats are spoilt or of lesser quality because of the light. **The best are walnuts, purchased at nearby farms, husked right before preparation of the dish or dessert, because the shell is the best packaging, far superior to any plastic.** In the shell the walnut breathes and is secure from external influences. In the future, most nuts will be sold in their shells, because the quality of these nuts is far better than those covered in plastic. **Only fresh husked walnuts deserve the mark 1st class.** Currently, the wrong system of labelling is in force. The whole family can participate in the husking, which brings the family closer together than eggs would bind dough. The tempo of life will slow down in the following centuries and once again family will be our first priority and society will be stronger. Still, in a different way than in the past.

Some people don't eat apples or walnuts other than in pastries and cakes. Finally, also they can enjoy something healthy. You can heat the strudels any time before serving in an oven at 50^{0}C, because the golden centre is protected by the golden baked dough. **We have accomplished a masterpiece, even the appearance is perfect.**

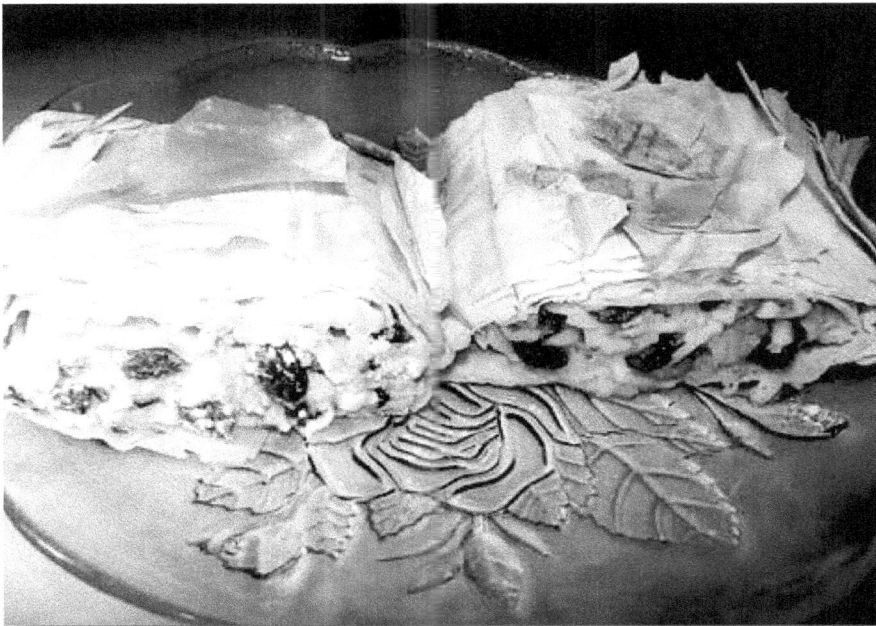

Dough made of sprouts:
200 g Kamut =
350 g Kamut sprouts,
cup of water,
honey,
salt

Apple stuffing:
2-3 apples,
50 g hazelnuts,
100g raisins,
honey,
lemon juice,
cinnamon

Banana stuffing:
2 bananas,
500g ground almonds,
vanilla,
cinnamon,
raisins

100 %
APPLE STRUDEL

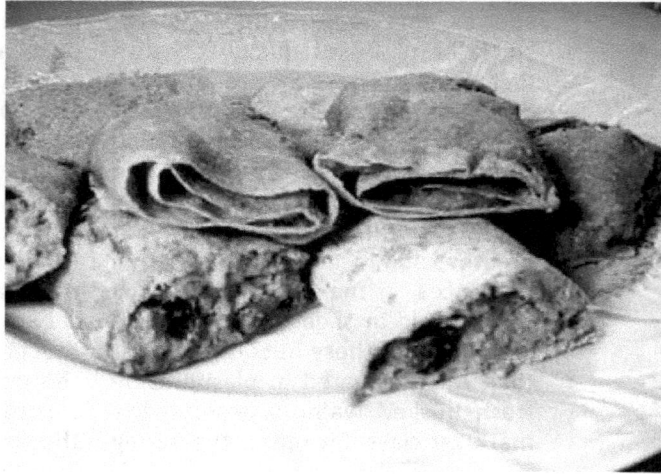

Three apples rejoice, as they are going to sauna instead of hell. They have tanned a bit, took a swim in refreshing water, they are giggling with the raisins and off to sauna in the evening. Gala, Jonathan and Golden Delicious. They will rise, but they will still remain fresh, they will perfume themselves with cinnamon, then off to the disco.

How to make a 'strudel' that doesn't involve an oven? Now, that's a little ridiculous. The apples are laughing, chatting and grinning. They're young, juicy, and tight and can do it all.

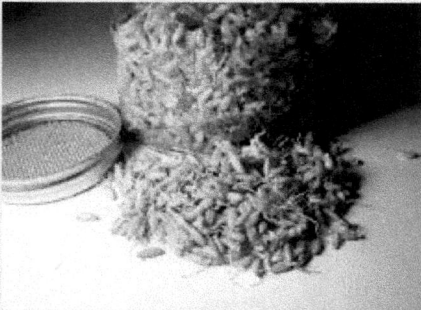

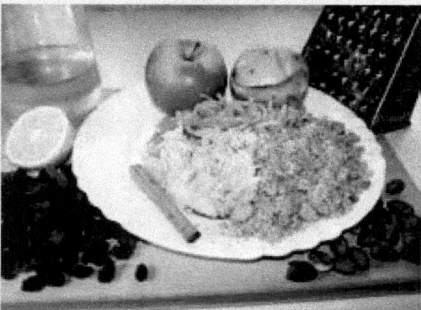

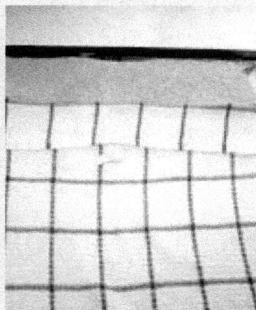

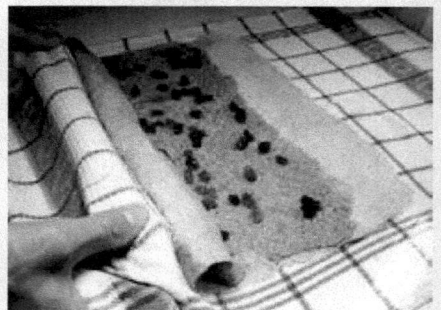

Blend 2-day-germinated Kamut sprouts in a mixer with a cup of water, large spoon of honey and a teaspoon of salt. **Spread the batter with a spatula on a drying surface to about a millimeter and half thick.** It requires some skill to evenly distribute the sprout batter to the desired width, but with a little practice a person can learn anything. In fact so good that later on this person can teach others how to do it. There is enough batter for four trays in a drier or 4 wafers. Dry them for a couple of hours. Use up the wafers right away, or if stored properly they can last for several weeks. There is a night and day difference between white flour dough and Kamut sprout wafers. The first is bereaved of essential elements, while the other is full of life. Sprouting namely increases the vitamin value by 10 times and more. Soften the wafer before using it by wrapping it into a soaked kitchen cloth. Spread the well-soaked cloth on the counter, place the wafer on top, now fold the kitchen cloth to wrap it in, so that almost all is wrapped, leave about 6-8 cm to peek out – this is the bottom layer of the strudel. Leave it in the wet cloth for approx. 10 minutes and carefully check when it becomes flexible enough to roll, but be careful not to oversoak it, then carefully place it on the dry cloth. This is critical part, than rolling the strudel is easy.

The apples are having fun, they've had peeling, and we've dripped them with lemon juice, grated them finely and coarsely, mixed with ground hazelnuts, 2 tbs honey and a substantial amount of cinnamon. Spread the filling on the wafer, sprinkle with raisins, hold the ends of the cloth with both hands and slowly roll it. "Bake" in a drier for 30 more minutes at 42ºC, slice and serve the apple strudel still warm.

The taste of the strudel is somewhat different, but the kids can have it as much as they want without fearing a visit at the dentist's, **but if you want classic apple strudel, which is still a million times better than the baked one, turn the page.**
Gala, wrapped in a blanket is chilling on the top refrigerator shelf from the warm summer night. Jonathan and Golden Delicious are on the slide facing new adventures… yeeeeaaaaaaaah!

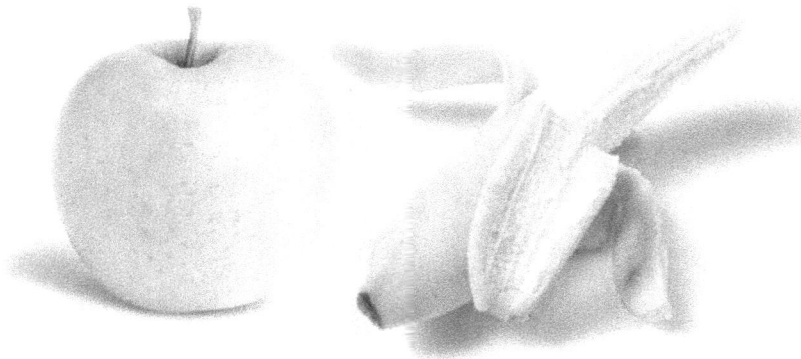

Natural marzipan:
250 g almonds,
2 tbs honey,
2 tbs agave nectar,
1 tbs coconut oil,
powdered vanilla

Chocolate icing for the marzipan:
50 g raw cocoa butter,
2 tbs powdered cocoa,
1-2 tbs agave nectar,
handful of chopped
hazelnuts to sprinkle

Christmas coconut balls:
150 g coconut flour,
150 g walnuts,
100 g almonds,
100 g 1st class dry figs,
80 g dry date nuts,
3 cloves of cardamom,
cinnamon, ¼ ts vanilla,
orange juice *eco orange peel,
a couple of drops of rum if desired

Royal coconut balls:
150 g coconut flour,
150 g hazelnuts,
100 g almonds,
4 medjool dates = 80g,
1 tbs honey,
70g cocoa butter or
5 tbs coconut oil,
5 tbs cocoa beans,
vanilla

MARZIPAN AND COCONUT BALLS

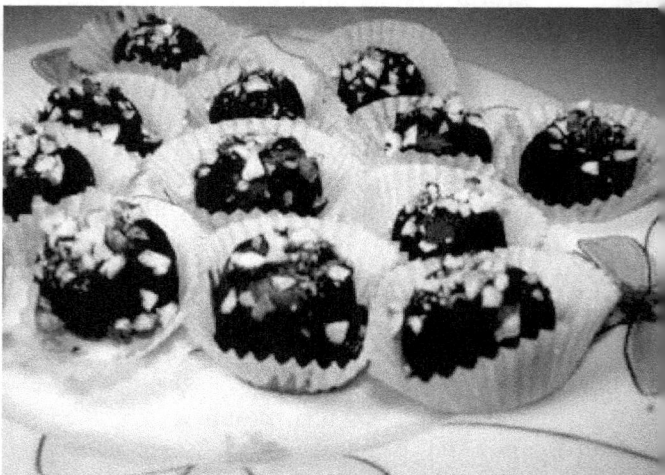

Life originates from life. A roasted almond has never sprouted, it is as though as dead. Almond is perfect the way it is with the peel and all. The nut husks and grain are the roughage, which the dieticians so highly speak of, so why remove them? When we destroy the balance by refining ingredients, we destroy the balance in the metabolism. Agave nectar and honey are for marzipan natural sweeteners par excellence, no white death and the doctor with a pill in the hand. I can barely remember how we used to make coconut balls out of

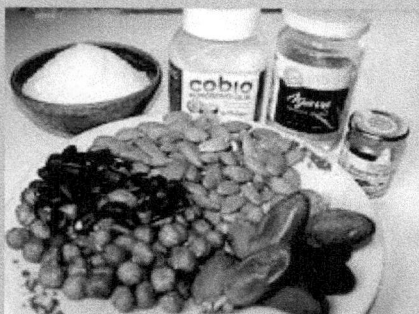

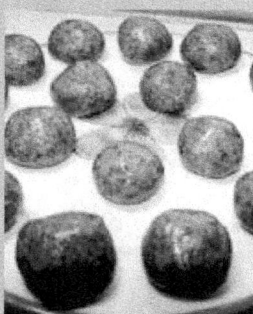

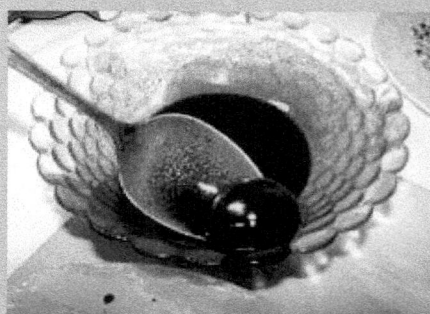

crumbled cookies in the old days. I can barely remember.

Grind the almonds in a coffee mill, add the natural sugars, coconut oil to make it more compact and vanilla for excellent taste. Make the marzipan dough without adding water; slowly knead the dough with a spoon – work those biceps. Form the balls and put them in the freezer for an hour, so that the chocolate sticks on afterwards when icing the balls. Make the chocolate icing as described in the recipe for moon chocolates and begin icing. **Fork the balls with a picnic fork and skillfully turn them when pouring chocolate on with a spoon.** The freshly coated marzipan place on baking paper. Sprinkle over with chopped hazelnuts. Yummy! **For those special moments...**

Walnut Christmas balls are a tradition. Grind a cardamom and cinnamon stick in a coffee mill. Chop up the dry figs and date nuts, soak in water sweetened with a little orange juice and after 15 minutes of soaking blend them into a cream. Mix sweet cream, ground walnuts, almonds, coconut flour, sweet spices and grated orange peel in a bowl. (A few drops of rum to taste won't hurt). Knead the dough, make the balls and roll in coconut flour. Bring the festive days on...

Imagine living in a wonderful mansion, surrounded by parks with blossing fruit trees and numerous ponds. Well, you're not the lord of the mansion, not the king, you are the main cook. Perhaps it was a mistake and you were mistaken as a baby with the fat guy...

If you managed the mansion, I mean if you were the main cook... Could you make the king coconut balls? People, you are the kings and queens wearing beggarly clothes. Stop eating slops and leftovers, serve yourself some wholesome food, there is as much of it as you could possibly enjoy.

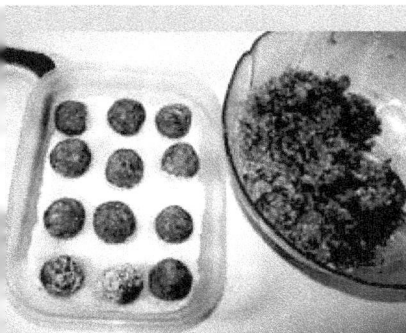

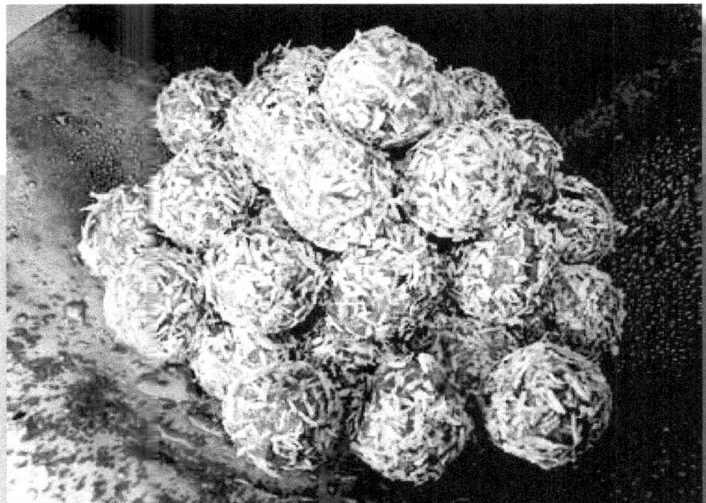

Napast orient:
100 g walnuts,
100 g hazelnuts,
100 g almonds,
100 g sunflower seeds,
100 g cocoa butter,
100 g dry dates,
30-40 g raisins,
4 cardamom cloves,
a small teaspoon of vanilla,
2 tbs powdered cocoa
for the chocolate layer,
handful of cocoa beans to sprinkle

Two cups of hot chocolate:
3 dl water,
2-3 tbs rice flour,
70 g fresh chocolate,
honey,
1.5 dl fresh,
unpasteurized – normal -
natural sweet cream,
cinnamon and vanilla

NAPAST ORIENT AND HOT CHOCOLATE

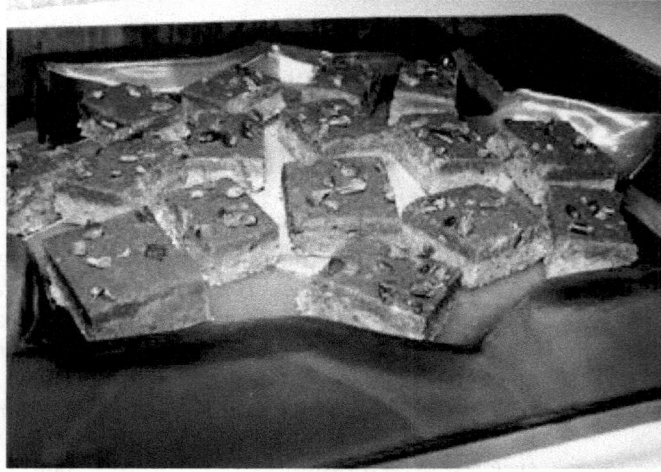

Napast Orient is the European version of the American fudge. My aunt used to send me her baked version, so I skillfully transformed it so it became edible for my standards. The first part of the name "Napast" (in Slovenian and Croatian language) is because it is attacked as soon as it appears on the table and almost instantly disappears. Hands with different colored finger nails hover over the plate and lower on the dessert as swiftly as airplanes in the middle of an airstrike. The second part of the name "Orient" because it can match the finest Oriental desserts.

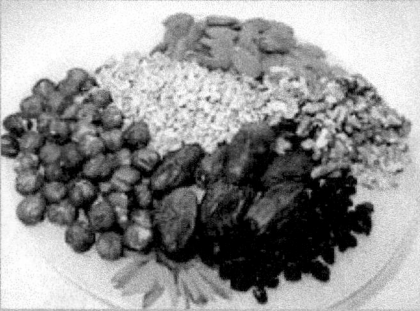
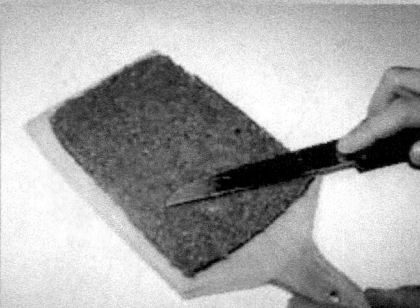
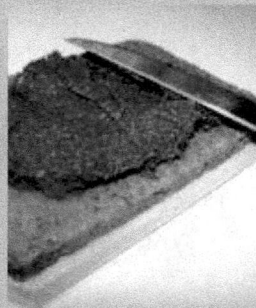
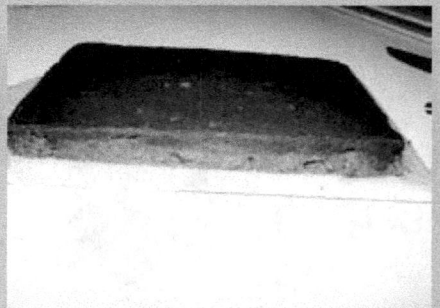

Grate the cocoa butter and melt in a double bowl or drier at 42ºC. Soak the dates and raisins for a quarter of an hour and blend into a cream with a blender. Grind the walnuts, almonds and hazelnuts, with a seed grinder and the sunflower seeds and cardamom with a cofee grinder. Grinder grind! ...Mmmmh, the scent of vanilla. Make the sweet dough and spread 2/3 of it on a cutting board wrapped with baking paper to about a finger thick. Best to use a spatula or cake knife to spread it. Shape a square half inch high. Place in the freezer for about ten minutes. In the remaining part of the dough, mix in powdered cocoa and place the chocolate batter on top of a double bowl, so it doesn't harden. Remove the first layer of a fudge from the refrigerator, layer with chocolate layer, sprinkle with cocoa beans and cut. Mmmmh!

Napast is similar to Bajadera, the original Croatian dessert from Kraš. Bajadera is an Indian dancer in a temple or funfair, someone in the limelight. Golden yellow beams spread like the sun rays from the centre on Bajadera's box. We hope that the sun rays also penetrate the laboratories of confectionery technologists in the big factories. The rays have already reached your kitchen.

Hot chocolate will impress those in love, the romantics and also the lonely, those on the look out... You will love the way it is served and enjoyed. You will only get the ingredients and mix them yourself. Sounds like tea for two, doesn't it? It can become a ritual like drinking tea. For two persons, boil two deciliters of water, slowly pour in rice flour and mix with a whisk. Boil for 2-3 minutes and pour into serving glasses. Let it cool, while you whip the cream. Break some chocolate bars on the plate and serve. Serve whipped cream and honey separately in a bowl. Hold the glass with both hands, talk some sweet foolishness and if it's too hot, lower down. Wait for it to cool a bit and try again until it's nice and warm. Slowly break the chocolate and keep eye contact even while mixing. A spoon of whipped cream...vanilla, ...mmmmmh, cinnamon....mmmmh, more whipped cream....mmmmh.

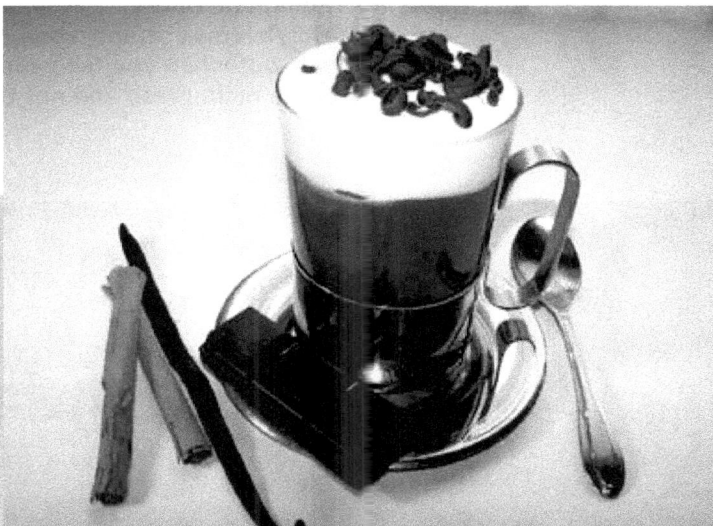

Kaki – banana – mango:
2 vanilla kakis,
3 larger bananas,
ripe mango,
2-3 tbs unpasteurized sour cream
or coconut oil for vegans,
knife tip of vanilla

Pineapple – kiwi – apples:
½ pineapple,
3 kiwis,
2 apples,
coconut oil,
honey,
cocoa beans

Papaya – banana – orange:
½ papaya,
3 bananas,
1 orange,
fresh chocolate icing

Mango- banana:
1 ripe mango and 2 ripe bananas
– blend and get the finest baby
meal or for those up until 99 years
or more, you can add sweet cream
if you wish to, fruit like grapes or
strawberries...

MIXED FRUIT PARFAITS

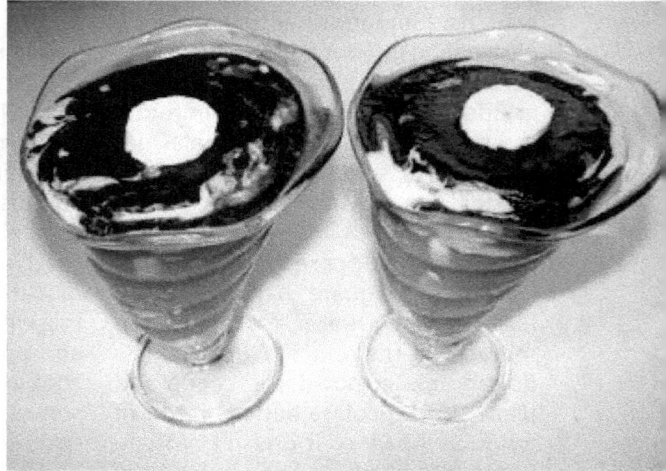

This recipe is intended to spread awareness of the scientific fact that fruit provides the main energy source for the body. **The human body is fuelled by fructose. Glucoseis the main source of energy for the muscles, it fuels everything in the body, gives the organs strength and revolves the thinking engine. Only fruit contains the right mixture of sugars for fuel. Our engine needs 50-60-70% of fruit in any diet, but, of course everyone can choose his/her own octane rating. All nice and well, but when you tell people that fruit is the main meal, and not the**

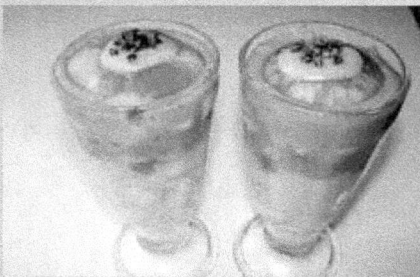

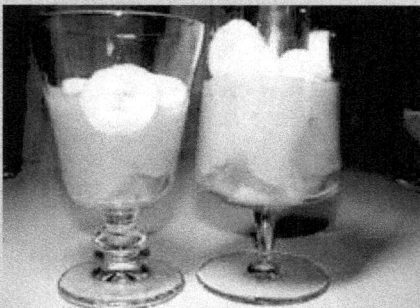

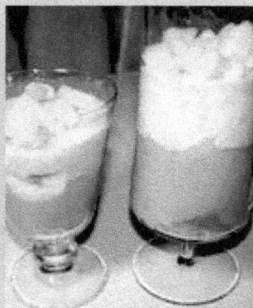

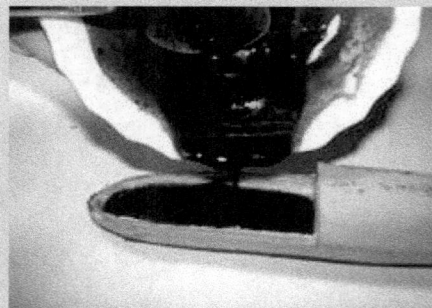

dessert there is no logic in this. It is the wrong education that makes us all ignorant.

A teacher stands behind the desk pointing at the board and explains while the pupils listen attentively: cars drive on petrol, electric motor on electricity, the human body on fructose and glucose. Fructose is the fuel, starch is the back up, because it is partially digestible. The fat greases the machine and protein renews the body. Fruit is the foundation of human diet; the dessert and the main meal, actually the main meal and the desert. When the institutions of the 21st century adopt the natural dietetic rules and the new generations are taught about this matter in schools, the glass factories will start making a new design of larger stem glasses. Everything is changing. Let's talk about one more mistake, one more problem, one more solution and finally the recipes.

It is wrong to think that mixtures of glucose syrups, inverted sugars, molasses, etc... as the products of the human mind can compare to the mixtures of Mother Nature. Only natural fruit juices on the tongue can stimulate bodily reactions, which completely absorb the sugars. **In the fruit there is a perfect ratio of various sugars - a mixture, which results in the correct breaking down of 'sugar dominos' followed by hundreds of subsequent chemical reactions.** In industrial candy, the 'sugar dominos' are scattered like being thrown around by a tornado. In medical books the absorption of sugars is listed under unsolved. Above is the basic explanation. Slowly to the solution.

The problem is that not ecologically grown fruit tastes bad and has little nutritional value. We don't have it enough, because it doesn't taste good and because fruit, which is ecologically grown, suffices only for 2-3% of the world population. We are lacking real food. **The problem is in the production, management and politics.** The solution is growing fruit trees ecologically. The best investment is when we plant a handful of stones or kernels, which grow into an orchard of bountiful trees. It takes a while, but the trees bring more and more fruit each year and your motivation grows each year. Two handfuls of stones to a millionaire. Start around your house.

I have revealed all the recipes. You can mix the fruit in a thousand of combinations. Fruit purée, fruit bits, vanilla cream, layer of another fruit, cream, third layer - make new rainbows appear in the glass each day.

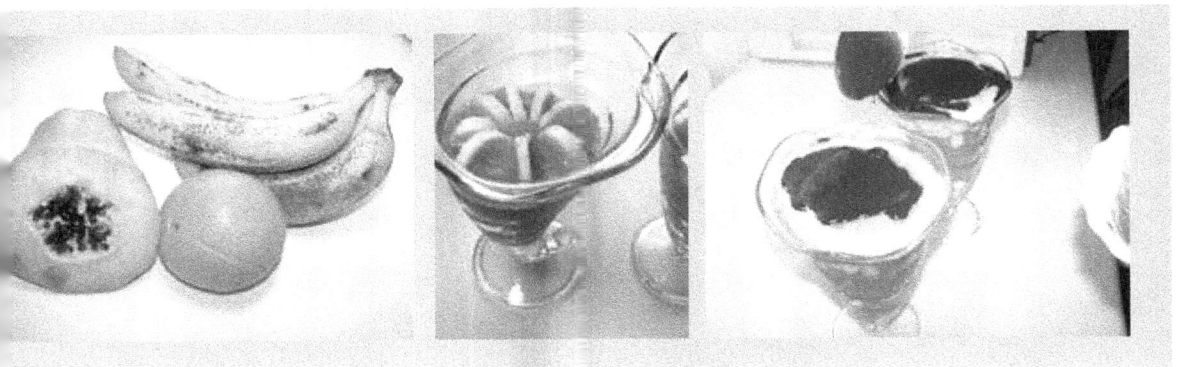

Vanilla cream:
100 g macadamia nuts,
1 dl cold water,
12-14 tbs cold pressed
hazelnut or almond oil = 60-70 g,
8 date nuts,
1 mini spoon of vanilla

Nougat cream:
80 g hazelnuts,
20 g macadamia nuts,
1 dl cold water,
12-14 tbs hazelnut or almond oil,
10 dates,
2 ts honey,
2 ts agave nectar,
4 tbs powdered cocoa,
pinch of vanilla

Peanut butter:
140 g raw peanuts,
60-70 g roasted peanuts,
12 tbs hazelnut or almond oil,
salt

HEAVENLY VANILLA AND NOUGAT CREAM & PEANUT BUTTER

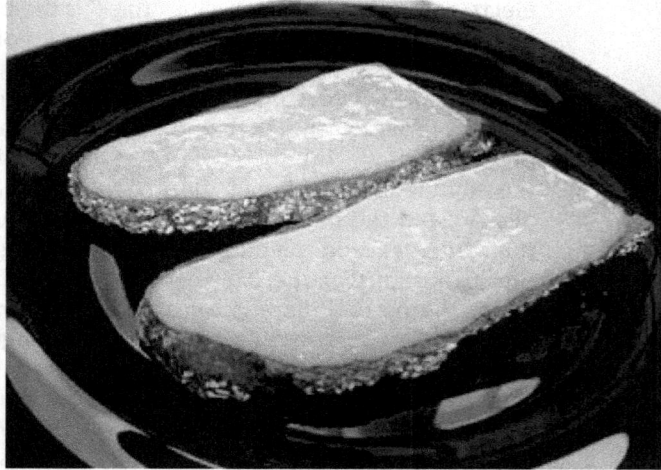

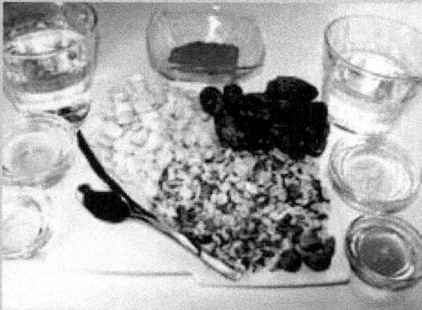

Do you believe the advertisements for healthy morning spreads? Some do and eat them every morning, the kids get sick, then the parents sue the sweet factory and, of course, win the lawsuit. There is not a hint of healthy in those appealing packages. **From a medical point of view it is pure poison. The industry of spreads will need some time for the health reform to touch them. In the meanwhile let's turn our backs on them and make our own healthy spreads.**

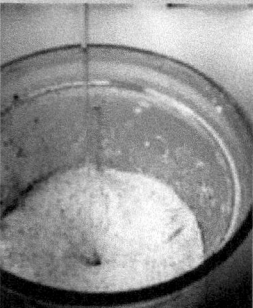

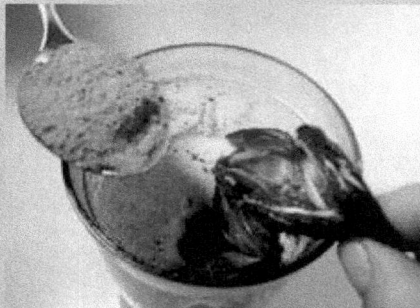

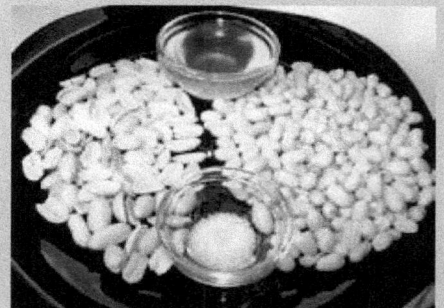

Chop the macadamia nuts, grind in a coffee mill and in a blender mix with water, until it is smooth and consistent. Use cold water which is a kind of water cooler, because fast spinning blades tend to heat the contents and the vitamins begin to disintegrate at higher temperatures. In the blender slowly add almond oil for the cream to foam and thicken, then add the dates and vanilla, and mix into heavenly good cream. **Stick to the order; first mix the macadamia nuts with water, then with oil and finally add the dates.**

Make the Nougat cream in the same way to counter the bitter cocoa, add an extra date, agave nectar and honey. **Use different natural sugars to complete the taste. We can keep the cream in the refrigerator for about a week.** The industry roasts the hazelnuts in order to make a really fine cream, but we can achieve almost the same if we dry the hazelnuts for a half an hour in a drier before grinding. The industry uses palm oil to make it creamier and easier to spread, but as long it is heat processed, we will leave it out. **When the sun reaches the vast plam tree plantations, we will enrich the recipe with a chunk of palm oil.**

Peanut butter is very popular in America, England, India and the Netherlands, whereas elsewhere only here and there. When I tried it for the first time, it got stuck to my palate, my tongue got glued to it and I felt I was going to suffocate. **A spread made of roasted peanuts and motor oil is suitable for the greasing** of machines, not for a human diet. Roasted peanuts taste far too bitter, but if combined with raw which are sweet, the taste improves and the spread is improved. **The specific taste of roasted peanuts mixed with mild, sweet, raw peanuts is simply worth gold medal.** The peanut butter is far better; it doesn't stick to the palate and proudly stands in cold pressed oil on healthy food shelves. Grill 30-35% peanuts for 8 minutes in an oven at 150ºC, then grind them together with the raw peanuts in a coffee mill, sift into a blender, add hazelnut oil, salt and instantly you'll have peanut butter all over the kitchen, on bread and elsewhere. Spread it in rolls, cakes, pies, pastries, desserts, toasts, and so on...

Future of sweet and salty spreads: Stone grinder as described in appendix of the book under title "Reforms". The big change or "Breakfast revolution" as I call it is very close to happen.

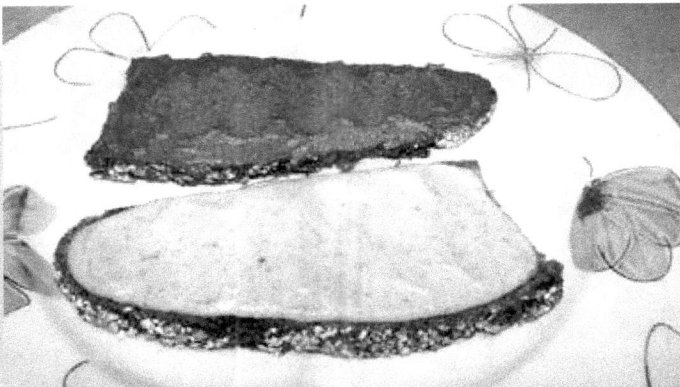

Basic filling:
50 g cashews,
¼ dcl water,
5 tbs coconut oil,
3 tbs agave nectar,
¼ ts vanilla

Black chocolate for icing:
50 g cocoa butter,
3 topped spoons
of powdered cocoa,
3 tbs agave nectar

Carob pods:
5 – 6 carob husks,
5 tbs fresh cocoa butter,
2 tbs powdered cocoa,
2-3 tbs agave nectar or honey,
handful of pine nuts to sprinkle

CHOCOLATES AND CAROB PODS

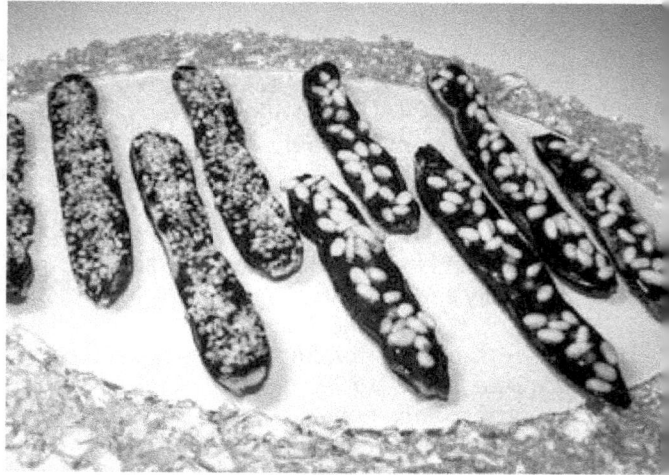

I am walking along the long line of aisles of different shapes, colours and flavors in a chocolate shop, but can't find healthy chocolates. The salesperson has never heard of healthy raw chocolates. During our conversation my eyes spot the sign: 'For your magical moments – happy moments.' I shiver, my eyes are blinded by the powerful light, I'm half lying down on my left; a nurse in blue is preparing an injection, on my right a dentist in white is starting his grinding machine like warming up a Harley. I awake from the nightmare and leave the store without buying anything. If I get chocolates as a gift, I give

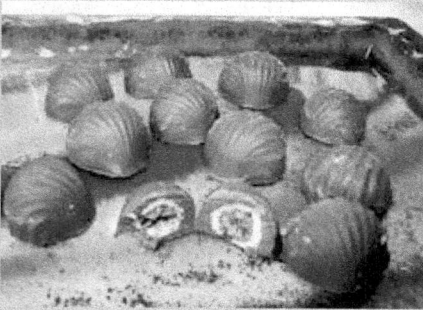

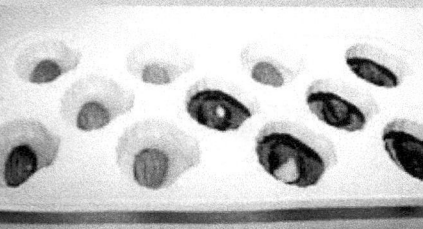

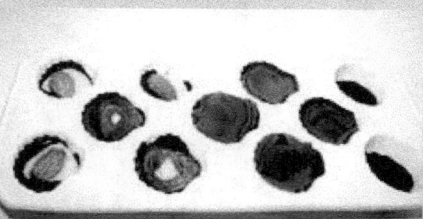

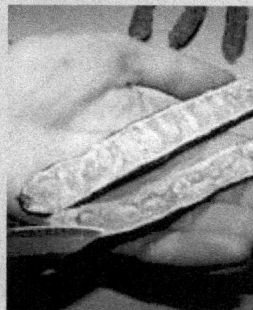

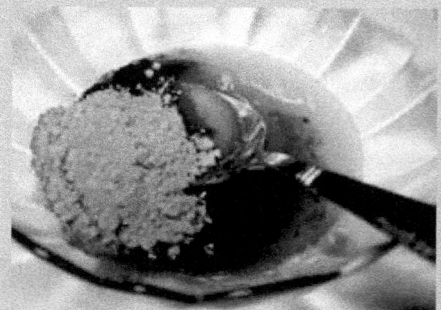

it to my pets. A lot of people would say that they are not healthy for a dog...

I look up far up in the sky and spot a cocoa nut in a treetop. I'm out walking in nature. I open the nut laying on the ground and countless cocoa beans pour out – this will be the centre of my chocolates, my nucleus. On the way home I gather some almonds and hazelnuts, cacao butter I have at home – I have all I need.

100% fresh chocolates will catapult you straight to Mars. On a scale from 1 to 10 they would be rated with 100. First we mix truly raw cashew nuts by using a minimal amount of water and than we slowly add coconut oil when mixing for the cream to emulsify and thicken. In the end sweeten the cream with agave nectar, spice with powdered vanilla and begin pouring in the chocolates. Use the chocolate models or ice molds, or even professional silicone models. Pour in the chocolates hearts up to a third or half, sink the hazelnuts, almonds, cocoa or coffee beans on top and leave in the freezer for a couple of hours to harden. Turn the mold upside down and push the frozen bonbons out so that they fall out. Rinse the mold with hot water so that the chocolate does not harden too quickly when pouring. Now we prepare raw chocolate pour it in a mold with a spoon until about a half of models, then sink the frozen fill into liquid chocolate, pour some more chocolate on top and the chocolates go in the refrigerator. This is one of the best recipes in this book. If we add 2 ts of coffee in the basic filling, we get dreamy chocolates for the coffee lovers. Those who don't drink coffee, try a full teaspoon of cinnamon. Whatever we put in the cream, is fantastic. We can fill the chocolates with vanilla and Nougat

cream from recipe 29. We can fill them with marmalades, which we jellify with agar. In the heart of the marmalade filling there can be a honey candied dry cherry, raspberry, blackcurrant, wood strawberry or another dry fruit. Remember how we intensified the aroma of the balm and mint compote – you can do the same with marmalade filling, before mixing it in. You can make healing chocolates, if you mix in one of the fresh super food powders that are so popular these days in the fillings... I don't think you'll ever walk into a chocolate shop again.

I'm walking on the beach under a tree avenue of mighty carob trees, watch the cargo ships and wonder how many containers of future problems will get loaded. I reach my arm up and pick some carob husks so I'll make some healthy cargo pods. Carob seeds weigh exactly 0.2g or 1 carat – useful for weighing gold and diamonds. The husks are for cattle food, you can get them in stores only around Christmas and mostly roasted and ground in flour to make cakes. A developed capitalist society.

The Bible mentions carob as 'St. John's bread' – so we can presume that once upon a time carob was the basic ingredient of a meal. Carob has a similar taste like chocolate, a specter of healthy sugars, loads of vitamin A and B, three times as much calcium than chocolate, less fat, lots of fibre and an abundance of rare elements. If only the manufacturers wouldn't roast it. Simply dry and grind it and the tables will be full of inventive healthy treats.
Split the carob in half with a knife tip, remove the diamonds, carefully load up fresh chocolate and sprinkle with pine nuts. The dog will be more than happy to eat the wormy husks, everyone has their own treat. Intriguingly good!

Pie crust:
500 g Kamut flour,
300 g raw butter
(for vegans palm oil),
1 baking powder,
1 tbs honey,
few drops of lemon juice,
a couple of spoons of water,
cinnamon

Apple pie:
700 g apples,
100 g walnuts,
1 tbs honey,
lemon juice,
½ ts cinnamon,
¼ ts vanilla

Blueberry pie:
500 g blueberries,
3 tbs honey,
vanilla,
1 ts agar-agar gelling agent,
2 dl fresh sweet cream

APPLE PIE AND SMALL GODDESSES

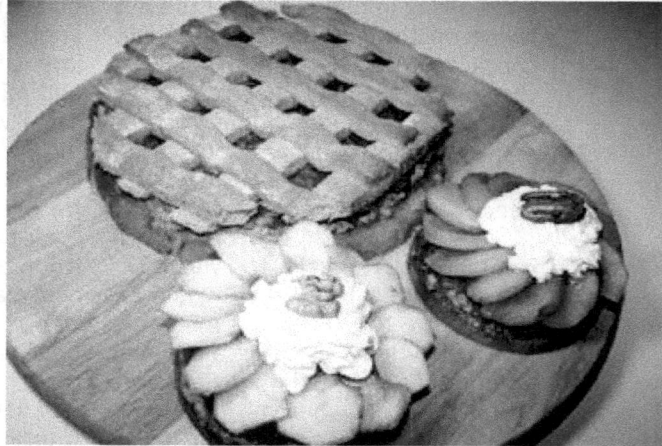

Name one person who doesn't love apple pie? It has even become an American symbol of welfare and a cultural icon. If something becomes a national symbol, you'd think that it must be good. Classic apple pie is not good for your health. God is crying when he sees housewives destroying apples in the oven and tons of white sugar with it. **In this recipe, we will only bake the crust and place fresh fruit on it and taste will be even better.** When God hears this, he wipes his tears and smiles. Half-fresh pie can truly become a symbol of prosperity and progress of the new world. Also pear, blueberry, raspberry, cherry, blackcurrant, peach, apricot and other pies can become similar goddesses.

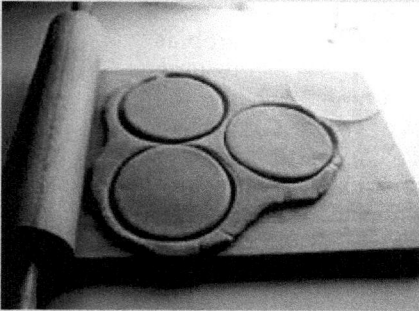

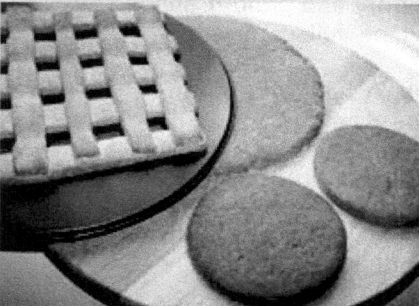

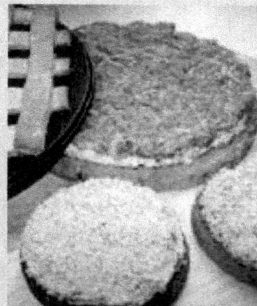

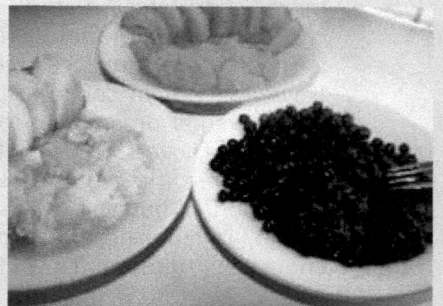

We will exceptionally break the rules of healthy food –by exposing oil to high temperatures, because we cannot make pie pastry without butter. Pancakes and pies are the only exceptions in our recipes. Sometime you have to sacrifice something in the name of tradition.

Make the dough from the above listed ingredients, roll it to about a finger thick, let it rest for a half an hour in the refrigerator, then place on a baking tray and bake for 15 minutes at 170ºC, depending on the thickness of the dough and the oven. Weave the net on a tray without edges, we will bake it separately. I prefer small round pies – little goddesses, which we carve out with a dessert glass 10-13 cm in diameter. We bake the net and little pies for a short period of time, around 12 minutes at 170ºC.

Grind the walnuts, mix with the juice from the grated apples and a couple of spoons of sweet cream and spread on the baked crust. Then follows a layer of grated apples: peel the apples, sprinkle some lemon juice, so that they don't turn brown, grate them half finely, half roughly, mix with cinnamon, vanilla, honey and spread on the pie. Place the baked net on the pie together with an even tray, where it baked and skillfully remove it, so that it slides off. Our golden core has remained healthy.

Little pies wear a crown in the shape of a spiral made of apple compote slices from recipe 13. If we opt for a softer apple variety, the slices soften as if they were cooked. Pear goddesses are excellent with pecans, scent grated pears with a mixture of cinnamon and nutmeg. Peach and apricot goddesses are without walnuts: cut the peaches or apricots to slices, partially squash with a potato masher or tomato and sweeten with honey. Add a thick layer of mashed apricots or peaches on the baked crust, to which we added the gelling agent agar-agar. Then make the crown from slices and a cap from whipped cream. In the winter, when there's no fresh fruit to be found, use natural compotes. **I named them goddesses because the crown made of fruit slices makes them royal and they also satisfy the royal taste.**

Also for the blueberry goddesses we partially squash the blueberries, partially leave them whole, marinate them in honey and of course add the agar. Something has to hold them together or else the blueberries would go for a walk. Boil the agar for 2 minutes in ½ dl water, leave to cool for a minute, mix with the blueberries, spread over the crust and place the pies in the refrigerator for 10 minutes. A bit of whipped cream and a string of pearls around makes them royal.

The blueberries have spread the word about staying alive, when going on the pie. They rolled, patted their backs, giggled and congratulated each other, the apple slices roared with laughter. Let fruit live to give you life, also in cakes and pastries. The American dream.

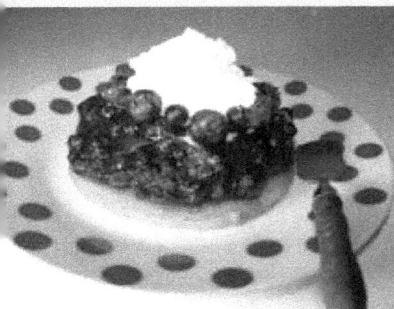

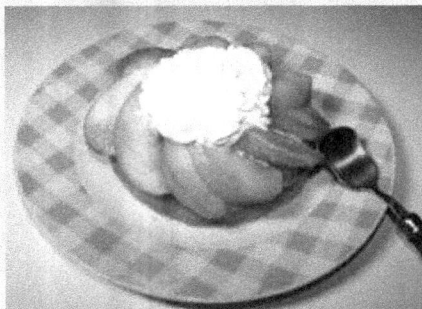

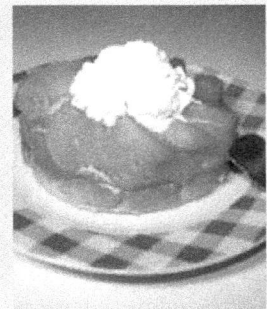

Potatoes for baking

Natural ketchup:
500 g ripe tomatoes,
60-80 g dry tomatoes,
½ red pepper,
½ onion,
4-6 medjool date nuts,
½ dl olive oil,
3-4 tbs apple vinegar,
½ ts cinnamon,
½ ts powdered paprika,
¼ chili pepper

Tartar sauce:
50 g sunflower seeds,
lime,
½ dl sunflower oil,
medium sized cucumber,
4-5 tbs sour cream,
½ onion,
garlic clove,
dill,
tarragon,
parsley leaves,
white pepper,
5-6 olives if desired

POTATOES WITH NATURAL KETCHUP AND TARTAR SAUCE

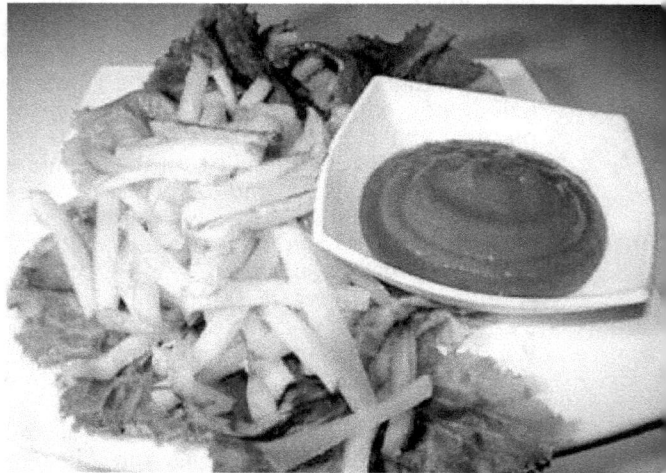

The McDonald brothers would love this recipe if they were still alive. This is a major step forward because the potatoes are not soaked in oil, instead there is a golden drop of cold pressed oil on them. What a difference! Baked potatoes bathed in healthy oil, served with natural ketchup or Tartar sauce can even become the symbol of healthy fast food.

It's so simple that you'll wonder why no one thought of this before. Peel the potatoes and cut like for your usual French fries, sprinkle on the tray and

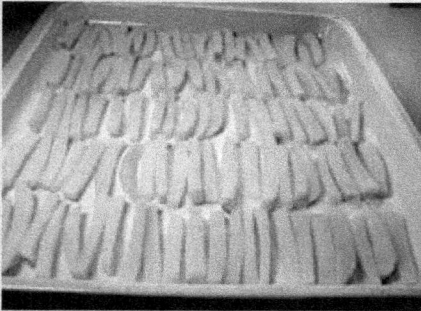

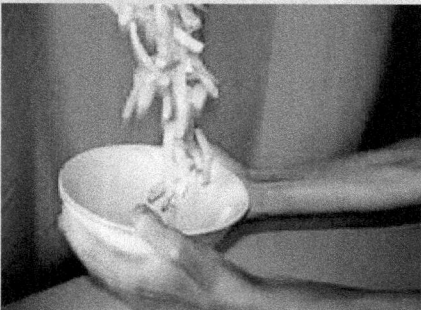

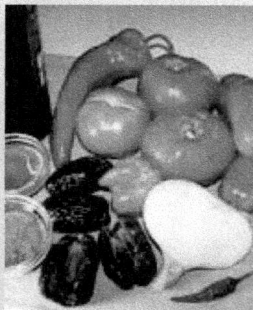

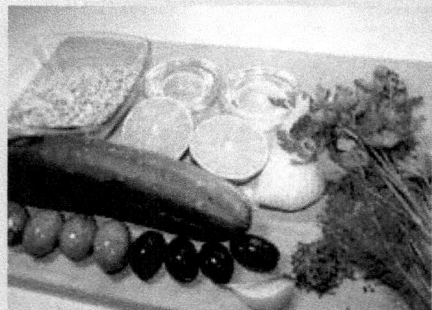

bake in the oven for fifteen to twenty minutes at 200ºC. Don't grease the tray, because we can easily take out the potatoes with a spatula and it will barely even stick. Shake it into a bowl, cool a bit and than drip with cold pressed sunflower oil and salt. Shake the potatoes in the style of the great cooking masters – with swift raises of the bowl throw it up in the air. Hooray! It is very good with cold pressed peanut oil. Now the sauces and we're done.

Ketchup from the supermarket is full of white sugar, overcooked, overly spiced tomato paste and a poor copy to the homemade ketchup. A billion dollar industry taking care only for money. Why copy, when we can enjoy the original?

Natural ketchup is spicier and smoother than tomato sauce in recipe 4. Soak the dry tomatoes for a quarter of an hour to soften up. Stop mixing and mix again in about 10 minutes, in this way you will get smoothnes we desire in ketchup. With a blender mix it with the fresh tomatoes, red pepper, onion, medjool date nuts, apple vinegar, cinnamon, powdered paprika and chili. Leave it again to stand for 10 minutes, then mix it until it's completely smooth. It has to stand for at least 10 minutes

for it to soften; an important part of the procedure, which we can't leave out. Although date nuts with tomatoes seem like a tasteless combination, it's actually very good. Medjool dates replace the sugar and gel the texture.

We make the Tartar sauce similarly as the French salad mayonnaise in recipe 9. Just follow the recipe carefully. Blend sunflower seeds, half a cup of water and lime juice in a blender. While this blends, carefully and slowly add sunflower oil while continuing mixing. This makes the mayonnaise creamy, thickens it and when the blades spin on empty, add the chopped cucumber, salt and spin some more. Shake into a bowl and finely chop the onion, garlic, parsley leaves and olives. A couple of spoons of sour cream, pinch of dill and tarragon and mix all the ingredients into a gourmet creamy sauce.

Serve the potatoes in a healthy style, on green lettuce leaves, with sweet chili peppers, cherry tomatoes and serve the sauce in a bowl, in which we can dip the golden potatoes. Dear mums, if you wish your children well, don't let them go to fast food restaurants! Dear gourmands, quickly get ingredients and get to it.

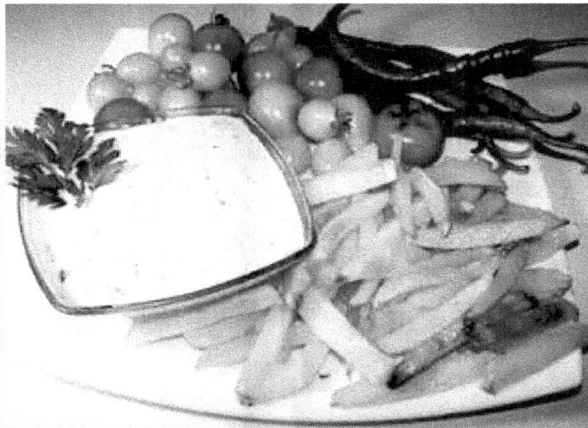

Corn tortillas or Kamut wheat pancakes:
250 g Kamut flour,
1.5 dl mineral water,
4 dl warm water,
salt,
coconut oil for baking

Spinach-nettle pesto:
150 g spinach,
100 g nettle,
bunch of parsley leaves, bunch of basil, 100 g fresh cheese, 6-7 tbs pines, 6-7 tbs olive oil, one garlic clove
Vegetable stuffing: avocado, sweet peppers, alfalfa sprouts, fresh grated zucchini, radishes, baby corn, different sorts of salads and sprouts...

QUESADILLA WITH SPINACH-NETTLE PESTO

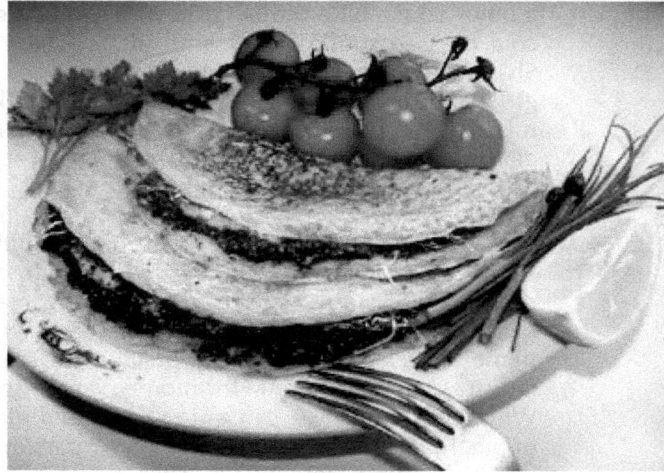

'   'Queso'' means cheese in Spanish, and together with "tortilla" it forms "Quesa-dilla", tortilla with cheese. The Mayas invented it, the Spanish conquistadors conquered it and the world adopted it. Quesadilla is not an only child, it has many brothers and sisters. I will introduce you with our healthy baby sister, who has never been on sleeping pills or sedatives, and never will. It is jumping around the pan like a lively fawn, it loves spinach, baby sprouts, nettle, pines and fresh cheese – and it adores Italian pesto.

You can easily throw the white flour

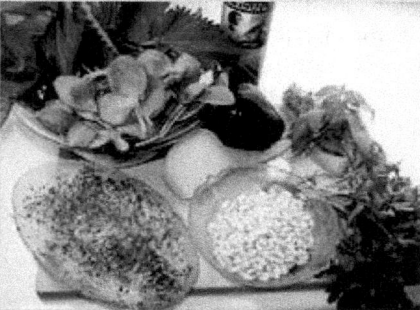

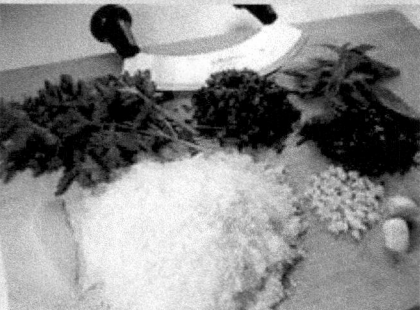

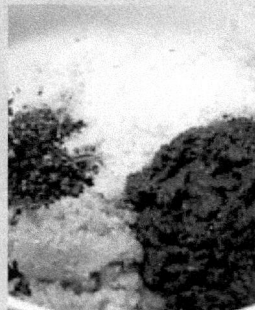

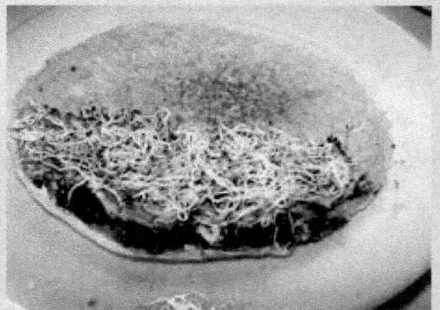

tortillas from the market into the faces of your government representatives. We will use corn tortillas or Kamut wheat flour pancakes and bake them using coconut oil.

The essence of our tortilla is pesto made from fresh herbs. Spinach with nettle and basil forms a very good pesto mixture. After this meal your level of wellbeing endorphins will rise above normal. The best are young nettles, you can pick them from spring to autumn, and they grow everywhere. They do not burn in the pesto and the civil engineers in your cells will be very happy to receive the iron sticks from the nettle. Do you know what a iron framed scaffold looks like? This is what nettle is for your body.

We cut the nettles and spinach, pour over a bit of oil and blend everything into a purée like spinach sauce. Finely chop up parsley leaves, basil and garlic and mix them with the purée with a spoon. Finely grate the cheese, grind the pines in a coffee mill or pound until tender in a mortar, mix all ingredients together and the great pesto is done. You don't have to add salt as the cheese is already salty or a bit only. Spread the pesto over one half of the tortilla, add fresh vegetables of your choice and fold them. You can fill tortillas with different fillings 365 days a year.

Why did we choose pesto for our filling? Because our digestive system finds it very hard to digest melted cheese and the cheese in the pesto is always fresh. Melted cheese slows down and complicates the digestion. Pesto is the solution. If every once in a while you really want to have some melted cheese, then bake the tortillas in a pan, sprinkle it with cheese and melt it separately, then fill the tortillas with fresh vegetables only when it is on the plate, as you don't need to destroy the healthy part of the dish.

Most of the meals can be prepared in a healthier way. **I want to show you that you can do almost anything, how to do it and encourage you to do it.** If you cook only the things you cannot consume in its raw state and prepare everything else naturally, you will receive the title "Master of natural cooking". You can thrill many of quesadillas' brothers and sisters for a healthier life-style as almost any can be improved, just leave the stubborn ones alone. Don't worry if something cannot be done, your menu is royal.

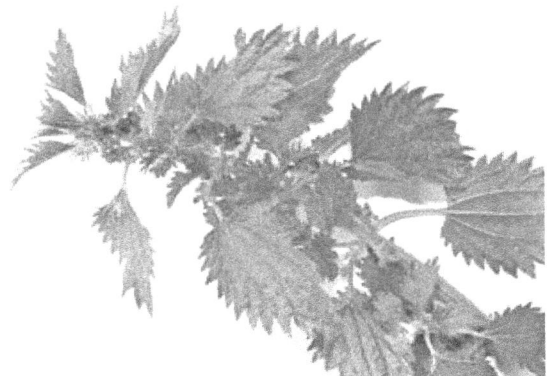

5 l pickled cucumbers:
2 kg cucumbers for pickling,
approx. 5 dl apple vinegar,
approx. 1 l boiled water,
2 ts of salt,
black pepper,
dill,
whole cumin seeds

5 l pickled paprika:
1.5 kg paprika,
approx. 7 dl apple vinegar,
approx. 1.5 l boiled water,
2 ts of salt,
black peppercorn

5 l of mixed salad:
750 g cauliflower,
750 g broccoli,
400 g carrot,
400 g onion,
approx. 5 dl apple vinegar,
approx. 1 l boiled water,
2 ts of salt,
black pepper

5 l of beetroot:
2 kg of beetroot,
several reels of horseradish,
approx. 5 dl apple vinegar,
approx. 1 l of boiled water,
2 ts of salt

2 l of mushrooms:
1 kg mushrooms,
approx. 3.5 dl of vinegar,
approx. 8 dl of boiled water,
1 ts salt,
black peppercorn,
bay leaves,
garlic cloves

NATURALY PICKLED VEGETABLES

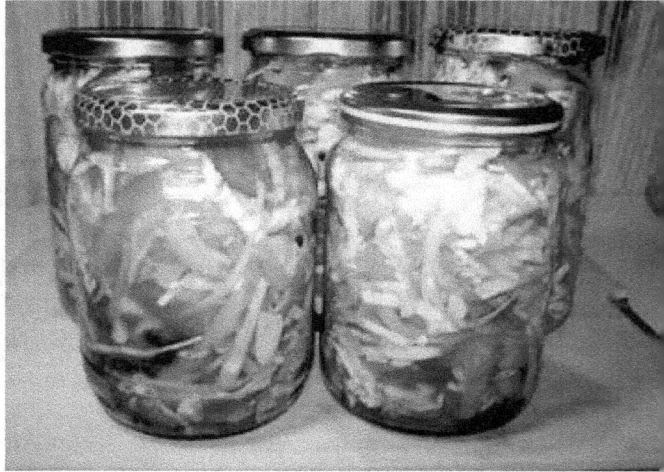

Mass pasteurization is a kind of a chemical war, but this time the enemy is invisible. Pasteurization is deadly, the ingredients in the food are instantly killed and people die much later in pain. The nutritional value of canned food is 0.0, because the temperature destroys the ingredients and then they stay like that for years. Automated conveyor belts are shooting out tens of thousands of cans per hour. It is happening non-stop with no intermissions all over the world. Home pickled vegetables, cooked in hot water are no better than canned food. The industrial processes for homemade canning or jarring has to focus on sterilization of equipment and glasses, not food.

Food preservation is an art. There are two conditions: food ingredients have to be preserved for a long period of time and their nutritional value has to be preserved as well. Honestly speaking 80

– 90 % of the nutritional value can be preserved, because eventually everything goes bad, and nothing can really match fresh vegetables. **There is no magic, just the good old, well-known preservatives: vinegar, salt, black pepper and strict hygiene. Vinegar does not allow some species of bacteria and fungi to live, salt prevents the off-spring of others, pepper is disliked by the third, and most colonies hate hygiene. The only difference is that we don't heat the vegetables...**

Thoroughly wash the bottles and sterilize them for 15 min at 120ºC. Wash the vegetables well and pickle them cut into small pieces or whole with a mixture of vinegar and water at a ratio of 3 – 3.5 dl of vinegar to about 7 dl of water. We prefer apple vinegar, because it has medicinal properties. Water should be boiled and cooled when mixing it with vinegar. As you can see, only glasses and water are sterilized and we put fresh vegetables into the glasses. **Time and vinegar will soften the vegetables in the same way as cooking would. And that is it. Shelf life of such pickled vegetables is not 2 years, but is just right at about a few months over the winter if hygiene was high.**

Pickled vegetables can be drained and served like fresh salad; pour over a bit of cold pressed oil and add a little bit of honey to balance the acidity. Every vegetable contains sugars, but when they are left in vinegar for longer periods of time, they get soaked with acid taste and that's why we need a small amount of natural sugar.

A few other instructions before I leave the kitchen bunker. Cucumbers can be pickled whole or cut lengthwise and they love the company of dill and cumin. Paprika prefers to be alone, cut into eight pieces with black pepper standing on guard. Broccoli and cauliflower in the third recipe should be grated, carrots cut to small sticks and onions cut into rings. The widow beetroot has found a new love – horseradish. If there is nothing else, run through the woods and pick some mushrooms, pickle them with bay leaves as a symbol of victory to come.

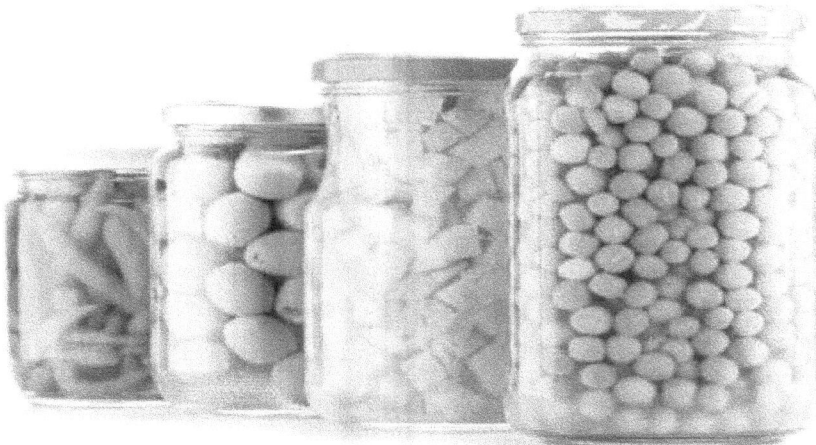

Sandwich with ajvar and eggplant:
whole-wheat bagel,
natural ajvar from recipe no. 7,
broccoli and mungo sprouts,
a slice or two of fresh cheese,
a couple of leaves
of spinach or lettuce,
a slice of grilled eggplant,
natural mayonnaise
from recipe no. 9

**Sandwich with avocado,
artichokes and oyster mushrooms:**
whole-wheat bagel,
squashed avocado,
broccoli,
mungo or alfalfa sprouts,
tomato slice,
cucumber,
2 horse radishes,
1 artichoke,
1 oyster mushroom grilled
and marinated in oil,
natural ketchup from recipe no. 33

Skewers:
seitan,
tofu,
ripe sheep cheese,
white goat cheese,
mushrooms,
vegetarian sausages,
cherry and date tomatoes,
cucumbers,
paprika,
sweet peppers,
spring onions,
zucchini,

SANDWICHES AND BBC SKEWERS

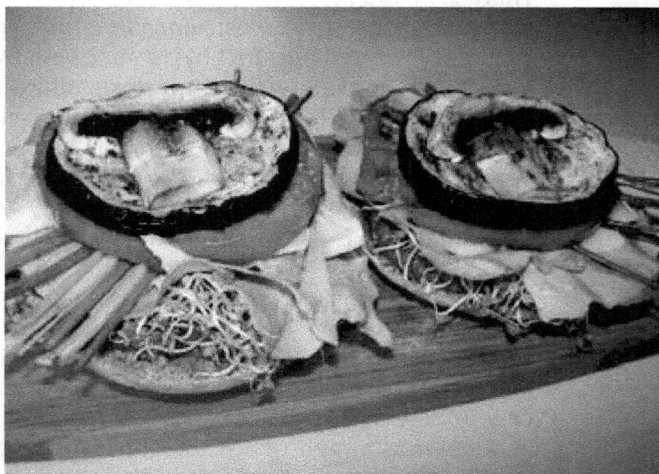

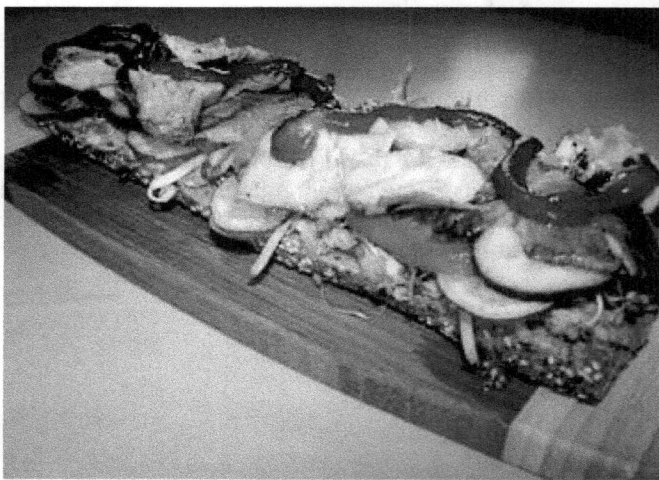

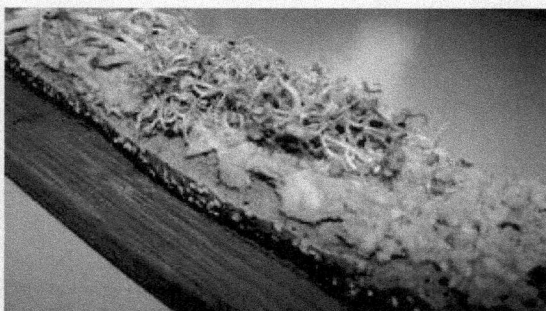

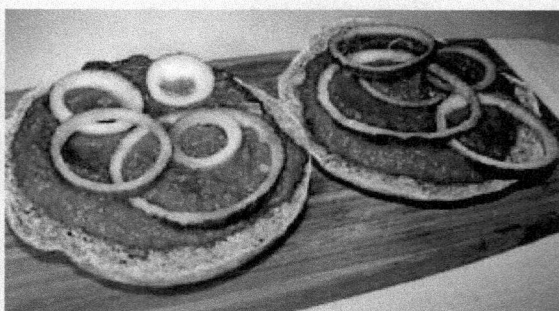

The declarations of ingredients and calorie intake in fast food restaurants, which were recently adopted in the American health reform don't change much, if anything – the ingredients have to change. The sandwich recipe is intended for the political circle, the managers of fast food restaurants, owners of smaller inns and for sandwich lovers, of course. **The following recipe gives the guidelines for new standards.** Whole-wheat bread without additives instead of white flour, thinner bread slices and 20-25% more vegetables will make a big difference. Ecologically-grown vegetables instead of pesticides, mushrooms, artichokes or eggplants instead of meat, competing to make the finest meat substitute, etc. These are changes. Then mayonnaise from cold pressed oil, fresh natural ketchup, frequently delivered fresh cheese from raw milk. These are changes. Tax deductions for restaurants, which would introduce improved menus on the basis of carefully drawn up directives – minimum share of living food in sandwiches 50% - these are all changes. How to make the sandwiches you can easily figure out from the pictures – it shouldn't be a problem, we speak more about global changes.

The directives should be a priority for the government, but I have made it my business and have decided to draw up the directives for the modern fast food. Cooks and some world-renowned chefs will assist in the making of new menues and the end result will be a special edition of the Medicine of Nature titled: » **Healthy Fast Food** – a book for individual use and fast food restaurants, which will then be able to print fresh green dot on the red and yellow billboards, which will mark the fast food renaissance.

A beautiful young woman is standing at the grill, turning the tofu, seitan and fresh mushrooms from the woods. She's preparing a picnic for her family. The modern Barbie opted for a vegetarian picnic. She's aware of global warming and how devastating livestock farming is. She loves animals, but not on her plate. She loves life and wants to live a long, happy and healthy life. It's a perfect day. She's skilfully turning vegetarian sausages, smiles at her husband, who she turned into a vegetarian with masterful natural cooking without any difficulty, the children are playing with the ball. Everybody knows that they've made the right decision.

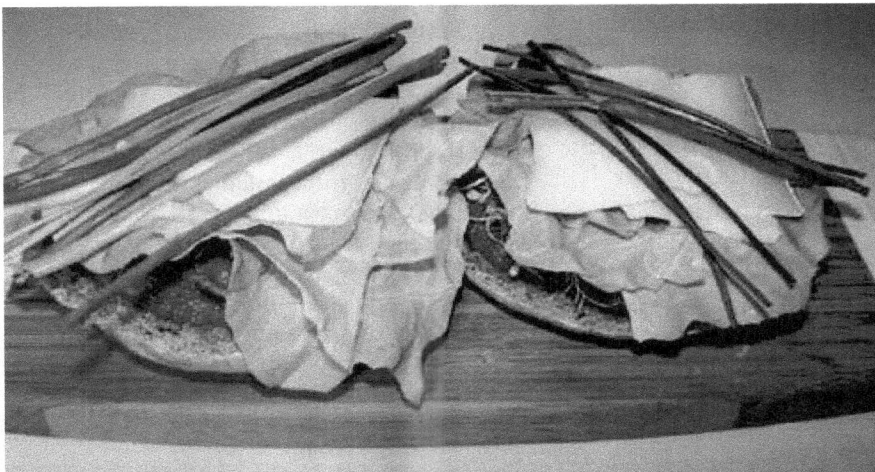

green and black olives,
capers,
radishes...
whatever

Marinade 1:
6 tbs of olive,
sesame or cannabis oil,
2 tbs of soya sauce

Marinade 2:
Marinade 1+ ½ ts
of powdered red paprika,
a bit of Muscat,
pinch of black pepper

Marinade 3:
marinade 2 + 2 ts of maca root,
2 tbs of vinegar,
1 ts of honey,
curry,
chilli powder,
2 tbs of natural ketchup or 2 dried
tomato halves crushed in a mortar
with oil

Tapas:
Fresh artichoke spread made of :
raw-fresh artichokes,
cold pressed olive oil,
parsley,
garlic,
salt,
pepper...

laden with:
olives,
capers,
cherry tomatoes,
onion, radish...
any vegetables

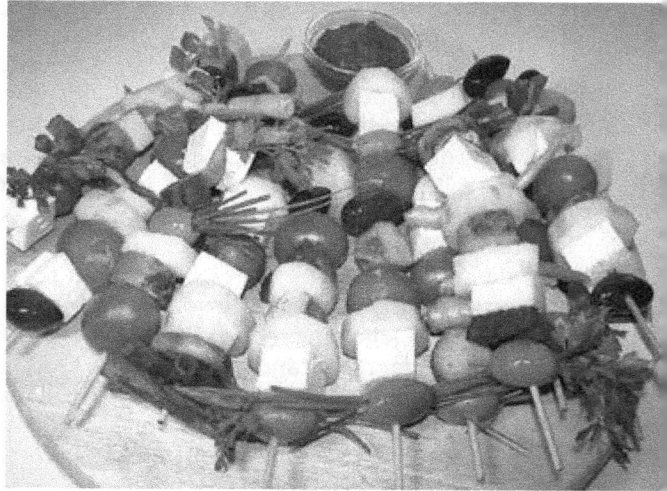

I can't imagine such a charming beauty with her kind eyes and good manners running around the forest with a knife in her hand, chasing a hog. Instead, she and her family went picking mushrooms early in the morning. In the fresh embrace of the forest, they filled their lungs with clean air, the most important human food, they got some exercise, talked and made plans for the next week. They came laughing from the forest with a basket full of mushrooms. A responsible woman and man !!!! knows how to take care of herself and her family. She has made the right decision for everybody. Let's see what they had and how they prepared their picnic.

The children have prepared bamboo skewers and cut cheese into cubes, dad had to prepare the marinade, and the housewife conducted the whole concert on the grill. When it got stock with the herbs, they smilingly exchanged their roles. The marinade has to be spiced with a feeling. Maca root is the so-called super food and its spicy taste finds its proper place in the marinade. Soy sauce is the queen of marinades and powdered maca root an exotic king.

Diced tofu and seitan were grilled without any fat, same as vegetarian sausages. The trio cooled down a bit and jumped in the marinade, where they scratched their backs every once in a while, and then put them on a stick. In between olives, sweet peppers, cherry tomatoes, radishes, fresh cheese were jumping on the stick... Strings of beads are colourful like the colourful necklaces on the aging ladies. We can stuff the olives with sweet peppers, pines, parsley leave, basil and so on.

Unfortunately, I have to admit that today's meat substitutes far from reach the quality they could. They are produced quickly from cheap ingredients and by using poor technology. **If the responsible governments would rather than finance space projects fund and invest millions and billions into the development of vegetarian meat, which is required to achieve a quality product at the level of a Mercedes, a lot of people would choose healthy meat, because the flavor and texture of vegetarian meat would equal regular meat and the price would be attainable.** I have experimented a bit with exotic mushrooms, but it is still in development. Technically with appropriate knowledge and technology one can achieve identical taste to any meat, but so far 0.0 budget funding has been invested for this type of solutions. Where do cancer and tumours stem from? Poor decisions about public spending.

Let me explain the term BBC skewers. BBC means "Barbie-Cute", cute as a Barbie. Beauty is a combination of external beauty, nice behaviour and most of all high moral values. Responsible men do appreciate external beauty, but nevertheless they put more emphasis on the moral values than women might imagine. I dedicate this recipe to the responsible modern woman to make the right decision.

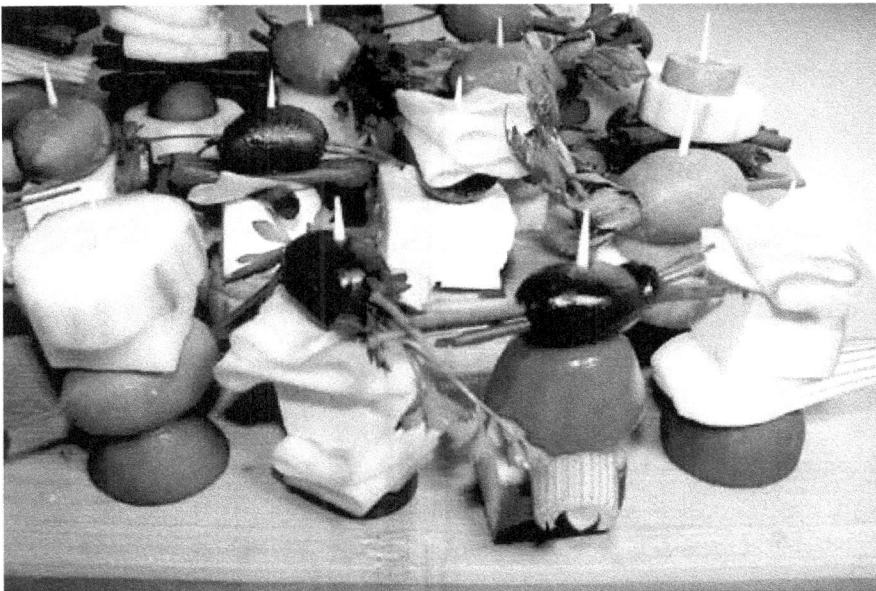

Lasagna and ravioli dough:
demand whole-wheat dough,
whole-grain flour and persist,
because it is your health,
which is at stake; until there is
another option, use whatever you
can get in the supermarkets

Filling for spinach
lasagna and ravioli:
500g spinach,
250g broccoli,
250g natural cottage cheese,
1dcl unpasteurized sour cream,
garlic clove,
parsley with leaves,
olive oil,
salt

Filling for vegan spinach
lasagna and ravioli:
500g spinach,
250g broccoli,
250g peas or 250g leek,
1 avocado,
parsley root with leaves,
garlic clove,
olive oil,
salt

LASAGNAS, RAVIOLLI, PIEROGY AND BUREK

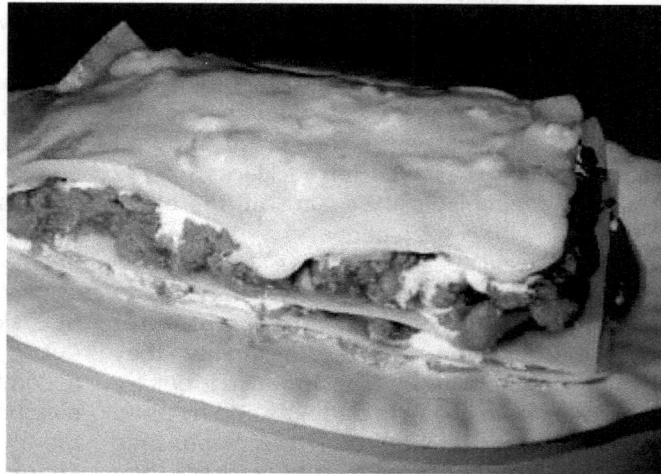

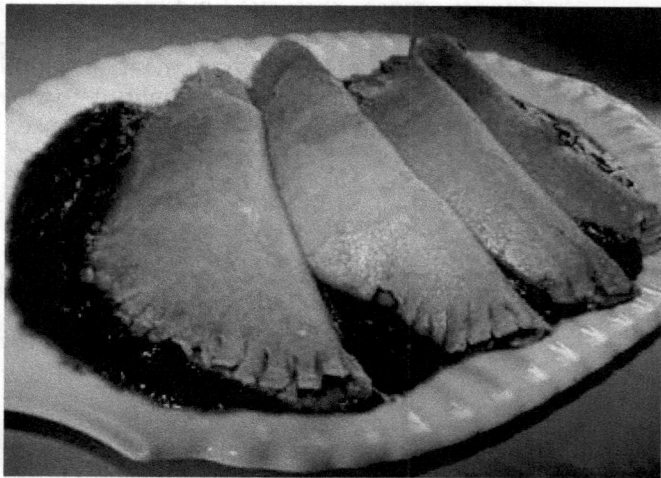

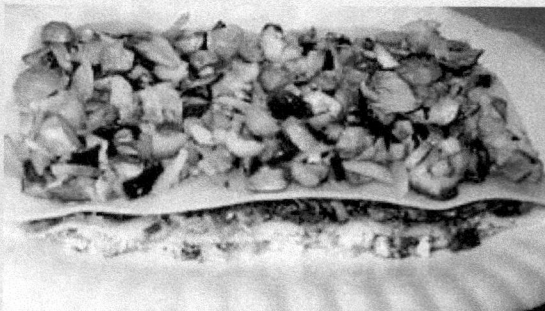

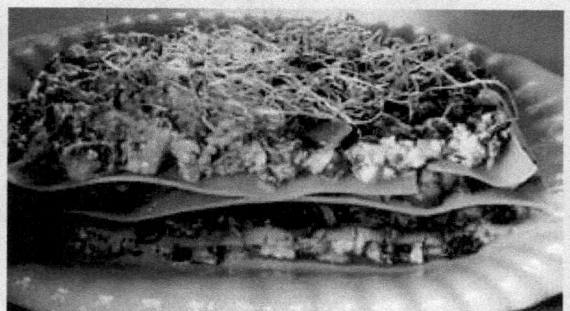

Lasagna is an epic dish, which was born in Greece, grew up in Italy and acquired its life education in the following recipe, where it lives in its mature years. Lasagnas, ravioli and other »rolls« are popular all over the world. People seem to love to wrap their food in dough. When I explored this culinary area, I couldn't believe how many different dishes are made in this way all over the world. One can barely find a place on the map that does not have its own specialty. There are countless regional and local varieties, but we will mention only the most important: "Empanadas and empanadilas" in Spain, Portugal and Latin America, "pierogi" in Poland, Czech, Slovakia, Canada and North America, "burek" in former Yugoslavia, Albania, Bulgaria, Greece, Israel, Armenia, the Arab Peninsula, "samosa" in India, "manti" in Turkey, Armenia and Kazakhstan, "spanakopita" in Greece, "pelmeni" in Russia, Belarus, Sybiria, Ukraine and Lithuania, "vareniki" in Ukraine, "momo" in Tibet, Butan and Nepal, "jiaozi" in China and Japan, Pasties in England, "maultaschen" in Germany, "ravioli and tortellini" in Italy, Europe and America.

All can be prepared in a healthier way. How? I will show you on the example of lasagna and ravioli, you can then make your local specialty in the same way, only with different ingredients and procedures, so you will have to rely on your own ingenuity and experiment. **The goal is to preserve 50% living, highly-nutritional food in the dish.** Cook the dough, bake it, grill it, whatever and then fill it up with a mixture of fresh and smoked vegetables, fresh cheese, herbs, etc. If some of this kind of dishes is not possible to prepare in half-half way (for example Mousaka) than serve fresh vegetables as a side dish in ratio 50:50 and your body cell's will be happy or at least they will not cry.

Cook the lasagna for some 8 min in salted boiled water and prepare the spinach in between. Roll the spinach leaves instead of blanching them. Place 2-3 leaves at the same time on the cutting board and roll them for the juice to come out and cut up the fibre parts with a few strokes with a knife. **Cooks usually compete who can preserve the prettier green colour by blanching, despite the fact that cooking cannot preserve the lovely green color. If you roll the spinach, you'll get the best looking green there is. Beautiful deep natural green colour, which will simply enchant you.** We will also soften the broccoli with a rolling pin instead of cooking it. First cut it into 5mm slices and then roll it so that the juice comes out, which is what also happens when cooking it. The difference is that in this

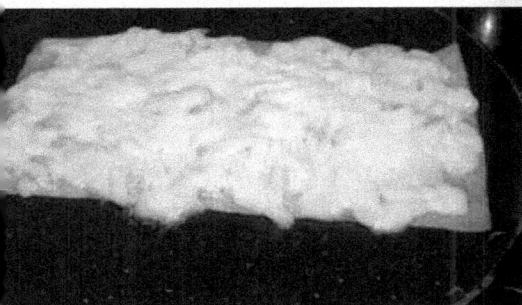

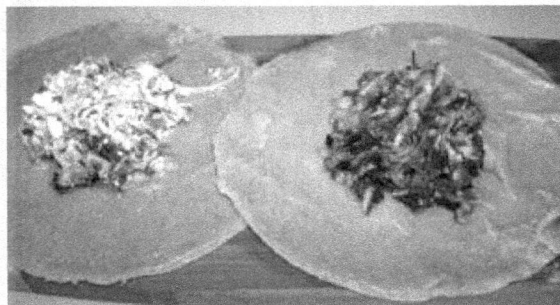

*Filling for lasagna
and ravioli Bolognese:
250g Hokkaido pumpkin,
250g mushrooms
or 100g soy meat,
1 carrot,
1/2 celery root,
80g sun-dried tomatoes,
olive oil,
garlic clove*

*Bechamel sauce:
2dcl homemade sour cream,
a couple of spoons of melted
homemade raw butter,
handful of ground sunflower seeds ,
½ finely chopped onion,
pinch of ground nutmeg,
white pepper,
cloves,
salt*

*Vegan bechamel sauce:
handful of sunflower seeds,
if we have truly raw cashews,
add them to smooth the sauce,
3/4 dcl water,
cold pressed sunflower oil and other
bechamel ingredients
mentioned above*

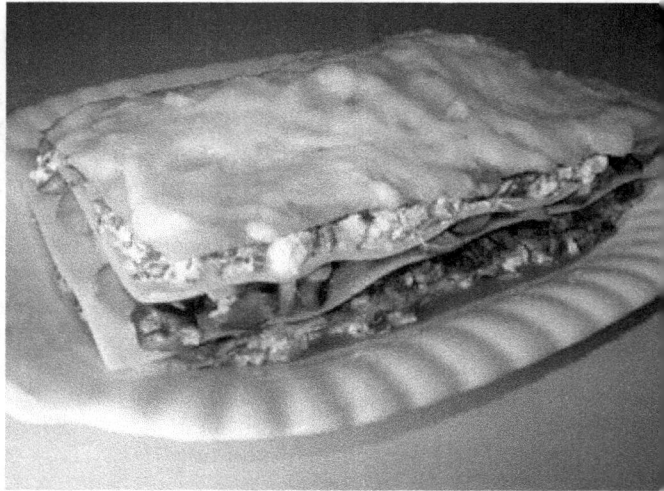

way the broccoli will preserve the noted healing qualities and vitamin C.

We did it, spinach and broccoli are soft, juicy and we have maintained all the life in them. Add the cottage cheese, sour cream, grated parsley root, chop up the parsley leaves and garlic and the stuffing for the lasagna and ravioli is done. Make the lasagna directly on the serving plate. Place layers of dough and spinach filling and sprinkle cheese over the final layer. Heat up in a pan or oven for the cheese to melt and you're done. We have a whole spectre of flavors, a perfect combination of health and tradition.

You start making the vegan filling also by rolling the spinach and broccoli. Instead of cottage cheese and sour cream we will add squashed peas and avocado. Cook fresh or frozen peas and squash it, baby peas you can only squash without cooking. You can enhance the flavor with leek. You can cook half of leek leaves and roll the other half and get the ideal combination between healing properties and flavor. Not only vegans will love the flavor, those almost vegans can try and sprinkle some parmesan to each layer of the lasagna.

Lasagne Bolognese is a super epic experience, one which even the Greek gods adore. Chop up ½ onion and blanch it on olive oil (exception to the rule). Peel the Hokkaido pumpkin with a vegetable peeler, slice to centimetre cubes and smoulder on onion by slowly adding water. Chop up the mushrooms and/or soy meat and braise for 10-15 minutes. This is the cooked part of the Bolognese sauce, now let's make the fresh part. Cut up the dry tomatoes and soak for 15 minutes, grate the carrots and celery and blend together with the tomatoes, olive oil, garlic and spices. There's no need to add salt, because the tomatoes are usually quite salted prior to drying. Mix the cooked and fresh part and make the lasagne layer by layer. Coat a layer with Bolognese sauce, then a spoon or two of Bechamel sauce, sprinkle with parmesan and repeat the procedure. Complete the delicious lasagne Bolognese in the same way as the spinach one with cheese melted in a pan. Make the Bechamel sauce from the ingredients listed above, why ruin quality ingredients? Instead of Bechamel sauce you can also put in a spoon of sour cream and sprinkle with parmesan cheese. Make a vegan version of Bechamel sauce from the ingredients listed above according to the procedure for mayonnaise in recipe no. 9.

Ravioli are easy to make. Cook the dough in the shape of optionally large squares or circles, put a spoon of fresh filling in the middle and close the edges with one of the utensils for the making of ravioli or with a fork. Serve the ravioli in any tomato sauce listed. The dough releases heat when cooling and heats up the middle to

the exactly right temperature for serving. There are countless varieties. Make the pierogy in the same way, the only difference is the shape. Cook approximately 10cm large circles and fill with the filling, fold in the shape of a crescent and close the edges with a fork.

The solution for burek is simple: bake the pastry in two round trays, 30cm in diameter. When the pastry is done pour over a mixture of cold pressed sunflower oil and natural butter, which saves the fats from high temperature. Distribute a mixture of crumbled ripe white cheese to the lower layer and a mixture of soft curd with a few spoons of sweet cream. The white cheese imitates baked cottage cheese, which releases water at temperature and hardens this way, but we use harder crumbled white cheese– an elegant solution, only the mixture has to be just right. Place over the upper layer of the greased pastry, cut to quarters and burek is done.

For other solutions, I invite you to experiment and discover new, healthy ways of preparing traditional dishes. The next cookbook Medicine of Nature is on its way, which will present traditional dishes from all over the world made in the maximum healthy way possible. It will contain a bunch of original solutions, even for fried dishes, like the Indian samosa. Are you curious? Let's check out the following recipe.

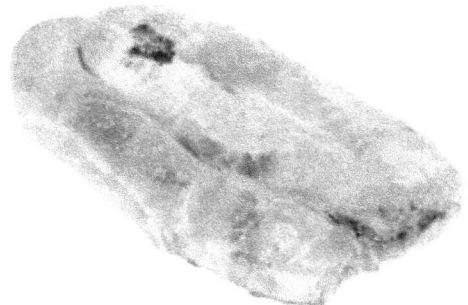

Potato dumplings:
500g potatoes,
100- 200g Kamut flour,
salt

Filling 1:
raspberry marmalade from dry
raspberries, honey and soaked
prunes or fresh raspberries dates,
soaked prunes and honey

Filling 2:
marmalade made of prunes,
blueberries and blackcurrant, fresh
raspberries or other berries
Sweet topping: raw butter from
fresh milk, agave nectar or honey

DUMPLINGS

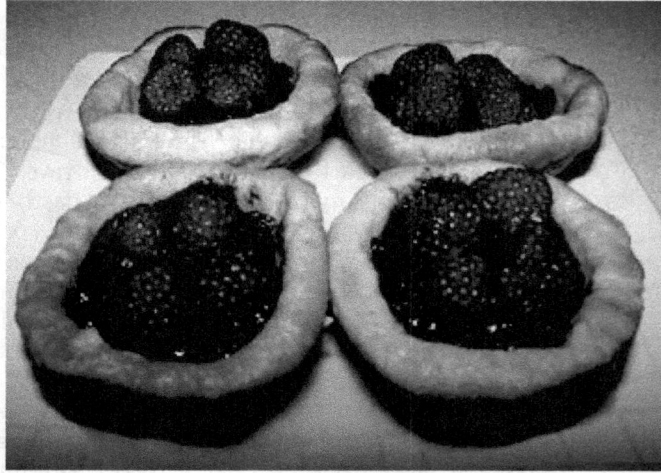

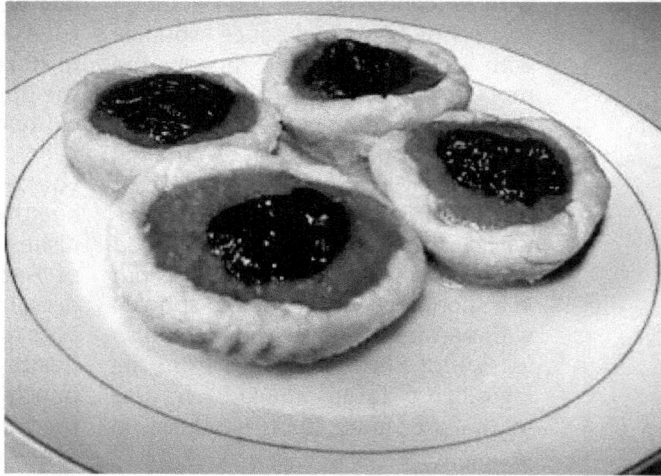

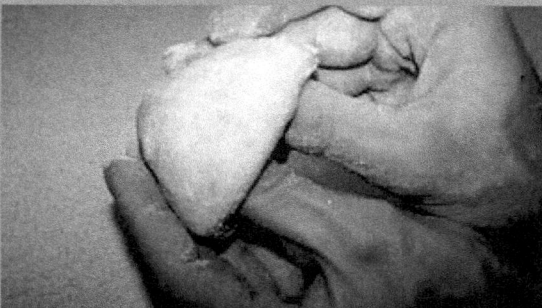

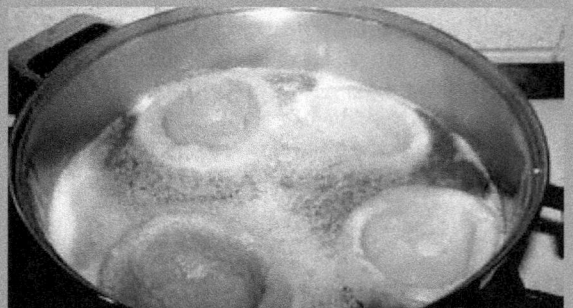

The most important food for humans is oxygen, O_2. The best restaurant for us is the nature: meadows, forests, mountains, fields, orchards, lake shores, sea shores. There's something in nature, which is missing in cities. We can breathe with all of our lungs. The open spaces are our natural environment and no matter how good the ventilation is in confined spaces, it will never come close to our living conditions, those which the open skies have to offer. Nothing charges up our batteries like spending time outdoors in the open air where the lungs fill up with fresh food, the body is invigorated and the biological motor runs on high gear. Spend as much time outdoors as you can, this is a valuable piece of advice. If you are fortunate to live in peaceful surroundings without noise, set up a quiet place on the veranda, where you can occasionally even spend the night outdoors. Sleeping outside 2 times per week from 9pm to 7am can change your life. Wrapped in a blanket under the starry skies you will have the sleep of your life and wake up feeling fresh and full of energy. You will feel completely different in the morning than usually and the fresh air will clear your thoughts, which is the result of spending time outdoors. The flickering stars will make you aware that the air masses are constantly moving and the movement of air currents accelerates and regulates the flow of bioenergy in the human body.

Another detail is worth mentioning. Namely, that the plants at night emit a different mixture of air than during the day, which you can sense during evening or early morning walks – the air is simply different. Sleeping outdoors connects us to the breathing of the planet, breathing of the plants, with our prehistoric life outdoors. Those without the possibility of sleeping out in the open air will find your solution in the nature project – the green belts surrounding cities, where you will be able to spend a weekend in idyllic little cabins in the midst of orchards. Medicine, gastronomy and architecture will be closely knit areas in the future, also through design and culinary aesthetic, which we will see in the upcoming unusual recipe.

Even in the world of dumplings, confined spaces are a big problem. Food wrapped in potato dough frequently complains about the heat, stuffiness, suffocating air and impossible living conditions. Prunes, apricots and other plums wrapped in a ball gasp and sweat for a while, but can't stand the heat. Still, there is a solution for every problem. **If we make semi-circles with a hollow for the precious content instead of balls, cook them and afterwards fill them up with fresh marmalade, natural**

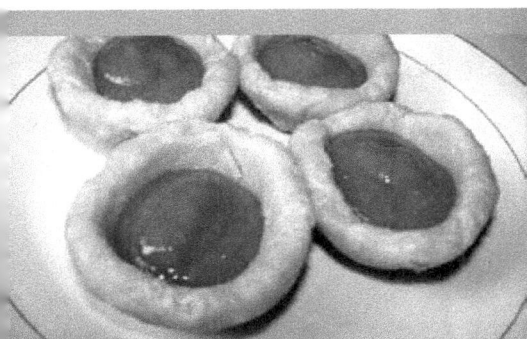

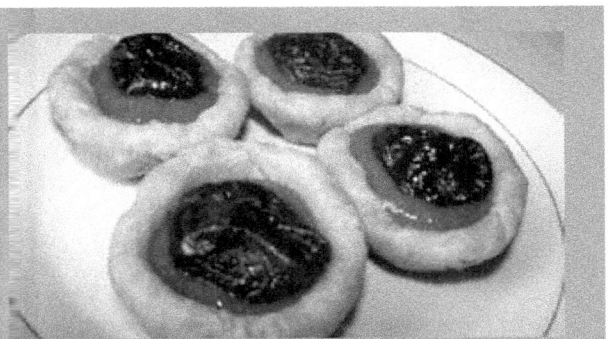

compote fruit or fresh fruit, we not only get a healthy solution, but an elegant culinary shape, which far surpasses its predecessors.

Cook the potatoes, squash them and mix in Kamut or other wholesome flour into compact batter. Make sure there is enough flour for the dumplings to keep their form in boiling water, but also remain soft. Make the semi-circular balls so that you hold a ball of dough in your left hand and slowly turn it, making a little indent with the thumb of the right hand. Once the indent is big enough, use both thumbs and slowly turn the bowl and shape it. The method comes from pottery – this is how they made bowls and cups before the discovery of the wheel. And still they do it in certain parts of the world; certain porcelain cups with incredible accuracy. The pinching technique, which is what it is called, is the first thing you learn at a pottery class. My first career choice was pottery, where I held also some classes, although back then I had no idea that these skills would one day come in handy in cooking, least of all in medicine.

Let the dumplings float in boiling water until they sink (10-15 minutes), cool them off and fill them with one of the delicious marmalades from recipe no. 2, dry compote fruit. Raspberry or strawberry marmalade with soaked prunes will enthral you so much that you will never cook the golden centre again. As far as apricot dumplings, let me warn you that dry apricots bought in supermarkets aren't worth a penny, because they are cooked instead of dried. Homemade dry apricots are heavenly and the difference is simply incomparable.

A glance to the future: dumplings in stores are semi-circular shapes, like little cannonballs, made of ecological ingredients, whole-wheat flour and there is a plentiful selection of fresh marmalades, which the manufacturers prepare and deliver fresh every week. A week is the minimum life span for natural marmalades. New frequency but healthy population.

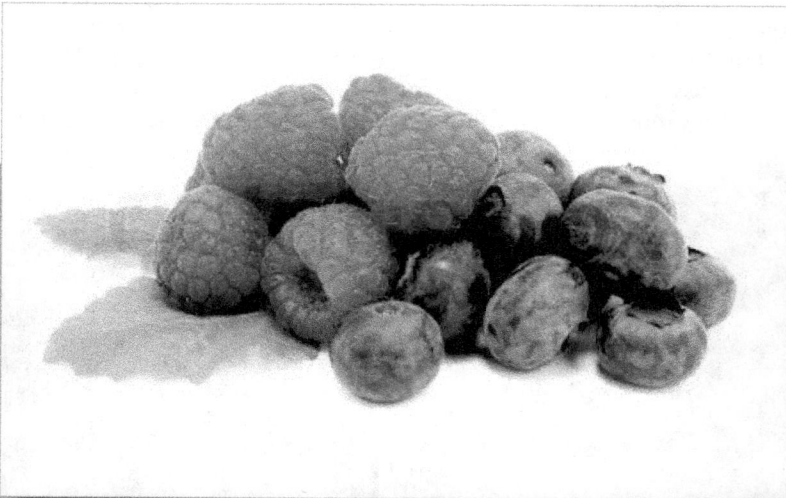

CHEESE CAKE

Classic cookie crust:
250g whole-wheat cookies,
100g natural raw butter,
2 tbs honey

Fresh nut crust:
150g almonds,
50g walnuts or pecans,
50g sunflower seeds,
100g date nuts,
a couple spoons of coconut oil

Lemon cheese cake:
1kg cottage cheese
from natural milk,
2 ripe bananas,
100g raisins,
a teaspoon of vanilla,

lemon glaze:
2 lemons,
10 topped spoons of agave nectar,
5 topped spoons of coconut oil

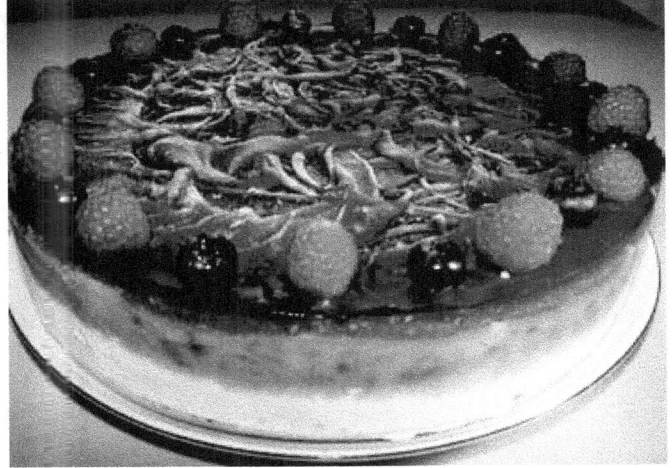

This cheese cake is so good and so popular that we won't waste any time and simply get right to it. We will need 6-8 litres of fresh homemade milk. Pour the milk in a larger bowl and let it curdle for about 2 days Skim the sweet cream in the evening and keep it in the refrigerator, we will add it back to the cottage cheese when doing the cake Wrap the curdled ball in a gauze and let it sift for two days. **Homemade cottage cheese is soft and tender like white clouds in the sky. This is how you begin making a cheese cake, not by baking the cottage cheese from pasteurized milk.** If you get the

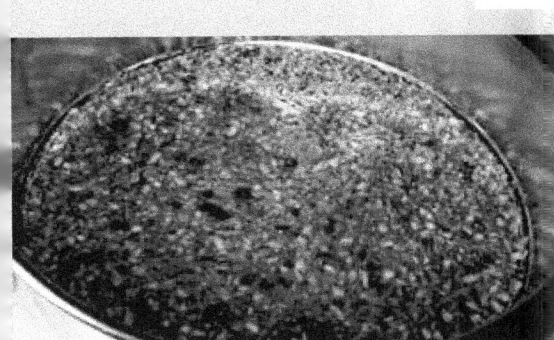

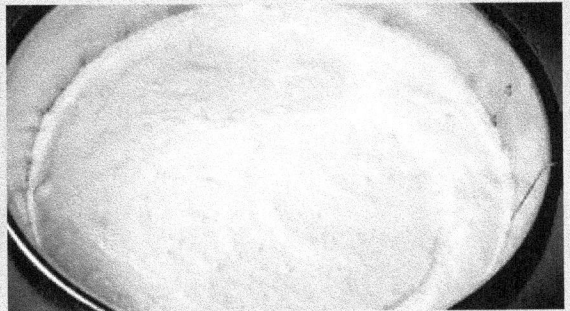

**Blueberry cheese cake with fresh
raspberry jam:**
*1kg cottage cheese
from natural milk,
2 bananas,
vanilla clove,
500g blueberries,
5 topped spoons of honey,*

Raspberry jam:
*500g fresh raspberries,
100g dry date nuts*

Chocolate topping:
*200g raw chocolate
+ 5-10 spoons agave nectar*

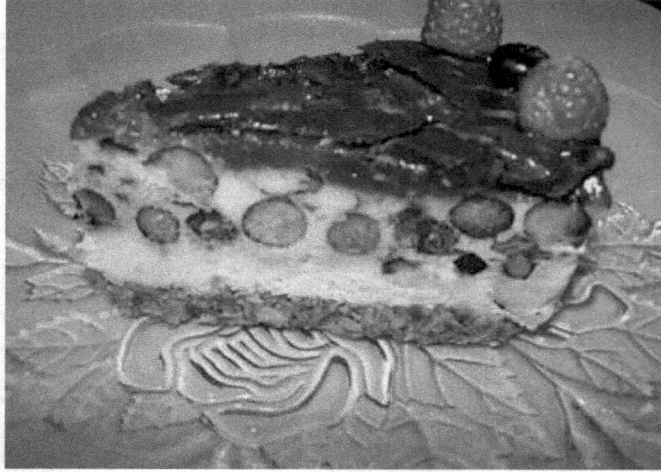

cottage cheese from farmers, make sure how much and how they heat up the milk. If they don't know the answer, they probably don't know what they're doing, the show the same ignorance as the governments all over the world. There is another way to find out what happened with the milk – before purchasing it, taste a spoon of cottage cheese. If the taste is grainy and plastic like polystyrene mixed with polyvinyl, better order fresh milk.

The cheese cake crust is usually made of crumbled cookies and raw butter. It's best to bake your own cookies from Kamut flour and sweeten them with stevia or buy a packet of the most natural cookies on the market you can find. Put a layer of crumbled cookies mixed with raw butter melted in a double bowl into

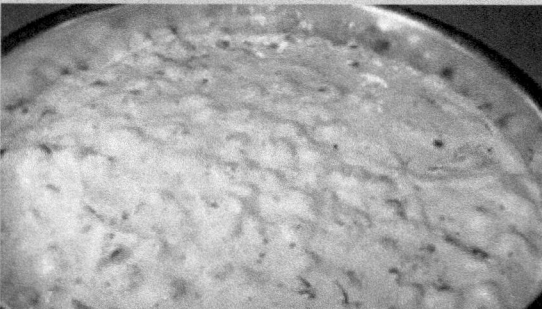

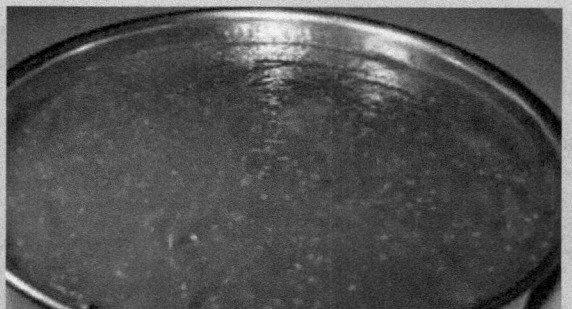

the model about half a centimetre thick. You will need a round model with a divided bottom app. 25 cm in diameter. **The first layer of cheese cake from nuts and date nuts is healthier, just as flavoursomev or more, but untraditional.** Finely chop the nuts with a larger knife, soak the date nuts and blend with the nuts and other ingredients. Whatever comes to mind, perhaps some cookies, some nuts or pistachios and coconut flakes...

Let's get down to it. Blend the cottage cheese in a mixer, add honey, vanilla.... Mix for a couple of minutes until smooth. Squash the bananas and mix them with the cottage cheese with a spoon not mixer. Bananas are great to use instead of eggs, they should be an eternal classic for the cottage cheese, because they balance the sour flavor of cottage cheese with their excellent composition of sugars and fibres. When the batter is smooth, divide it up into several bowls and add different fruit and extras and pour in the layers one by one in the model. Using a spoon, mix in blueberries, raspberries, soaked raisins, chocolate pieces or other fruit, depending on the recipe.

Now for the glaze. Squeeze two lemons for the lemon juice, perhaps a lime or an orange, add the agave nectar and melted coconut oil and pour over the cheese cake, maybe you will need agar-agar, experiment. A very good marmalade is made of fresh raspberries and date nuts or jelly from agar-agar and squashed fresh raspberries, perhaps strawberries. For the chocolate coating, choose fresh chocolate, carefully melt it over a double bowl, add agave nectar, which makes the chocolate consistency best for creating relief traces by pouring, as we can see in the picture. Freeze the cheese cake for a couple of hours, then store it in the refrigerator before slicing and serving this super dessert.

There are a million varieties for cheese cake, an internet query comes back with 390 million hits in 0.2 seconds, but there is only one procedure for the original cheese cake from now on. There are also a million and a million great ones, fresh and vegan recipes for cheese cake, but my task is to improve and revive the good old classic, which is used in 99% cases.

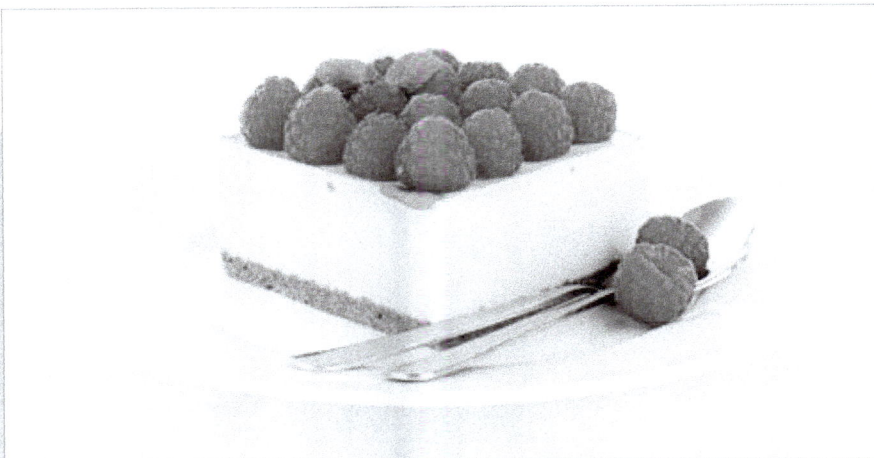

Spring potion:
1 kg apples,
100-200 g alfalfa sprouts

Green star:
2 slices of pineapple,
2 apples,
1 pear,
3 firmer kiwis

Natural Schweppes:
1 baby pineapple,
1 grapefruit,
3-4 dl mineral water

Pink dreams and Green Martian:
5-6 apples,
1 pomegranate,
sprigs of fresh lemon balm

Carrot juice:
Fresh organic carrots

Mango cocktail:
1 mango,
2 slices of pineapple,
2 oranges,
5-10 tangerines,
1 lime

Sweet wine:
1 kg apples,
200 – 400 g beetroot

NATURAL JUICES

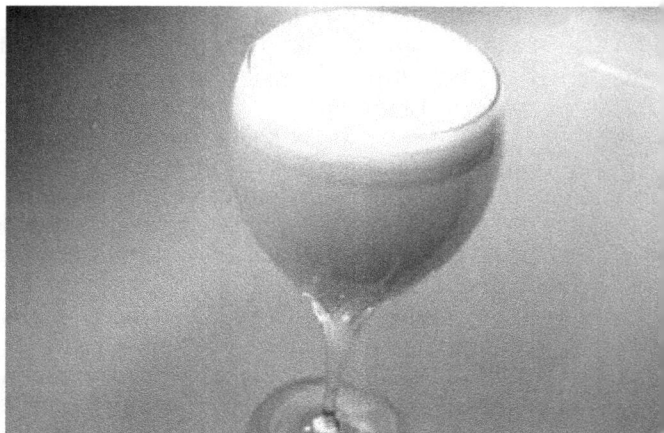

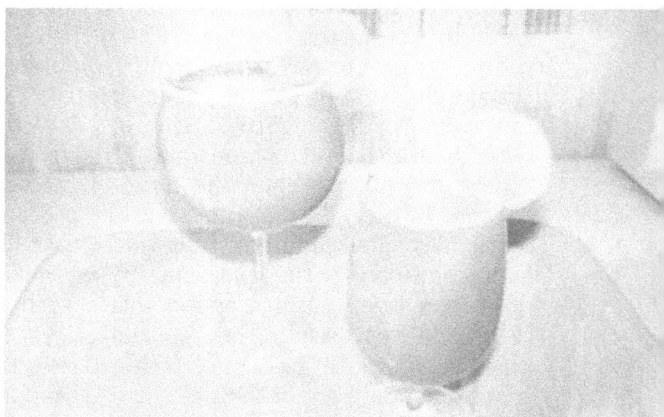

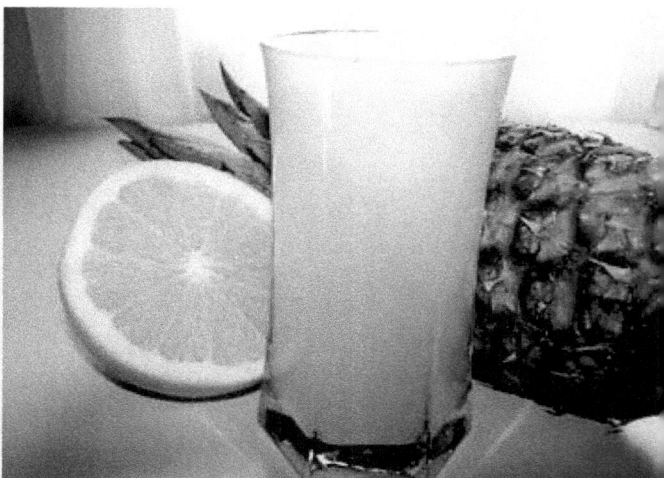

When talking with people from Spain, I discovered that in Spain freshly squeezed orange juice is a tradition. When I mentioned orange juice from a carton, they looked at me rather funnily, as if to say, if I'm OK. In certain, especially trop c countries, freshly squeezed juices are a standard, in most other civilizatior s the standard is pasteurization. Wrong standards. Sad to say but even in Spain, where there is aboundance of fresh oranges nowadays hectolitres of pasteurized orange juice are sold.

If the production of clear, thick juices and other colourful junk would be diverted to the sewage in the river, we would get a new Amazon river. Those juices have nothing in common with life, they are like rocks in the middle of the river – obstructing its natural flow. The stream of life is supported by living juices, which are the elixir of life. There are countless combination;, but the **Holy Grail that people have been searching for thousands of years, the cup of life hidden in the mysticism, probably belongs to the carrot juice or natural Schweppes which is sparkling heaven. The first one is best from medical point of view, the other from palatable point of view.**

Apple and alfalfa sprouts juice is a spring potion, essential when you are fasting or semi-fasting with juices. Alfalfa sprouts have the same effect on the body's recovery as the spring sun has on the plant kingdom. Sprouts contain youthful energy, the energy of growth, which the Indians would call the energy of spring.

Green star is the star of the winter. This juice got its name after the juicer Green Star and it well deserves it, as Green Star is an excellent juicer for great juices.

You absolutely have to try natural Schweppes! It is a very good body cleanser and provides excellent refreshment. Pineapple gives a sweet-sour component of taste, grapefruit makes adds bitterness and sparkling mineral water charges the refreshing drink with its bubbles. Half a baby pineapple and clean out the heartwood with a knife; squeeze the juice out with an electric

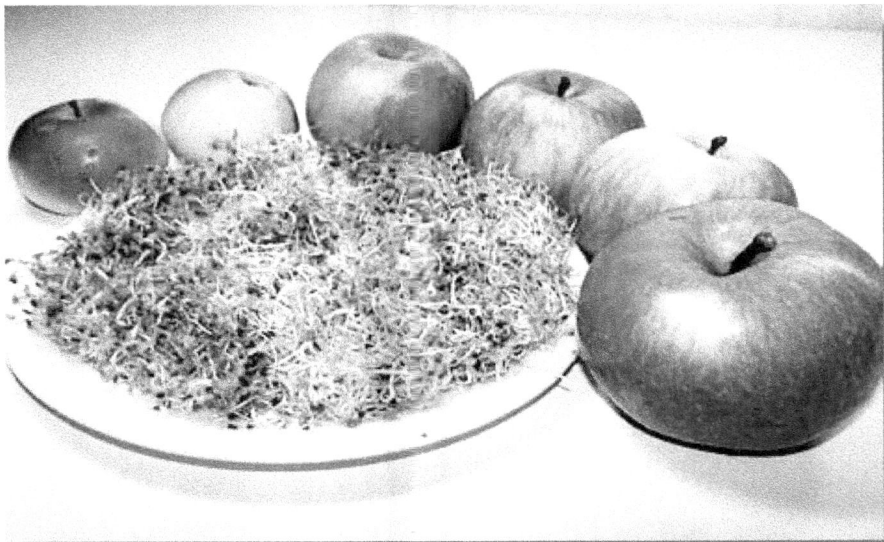

juicer and add some grapefruit. Strain the juice and add mineral water to taste. Ssssss... **Natural Schweppes is much better than the original...............................**
Pink dreams conjure up a harmony for the taste buds and a potion of vitamin C. Before granules of pomegranate are squeezed into the juice we have to get them out: cut the pomegranate in two halves and use the back of the spoon to tap on the peel so the granules fall out (tap pretty strong). Green Martian is juice made with squeezed apples and lemon balm. Use one larger twig of lemon balm per one apple.

Fresh carrot juice is one of the most universal medicines in the world. The healing potential of juice is measured by its freshness and organic production. Juice prepared

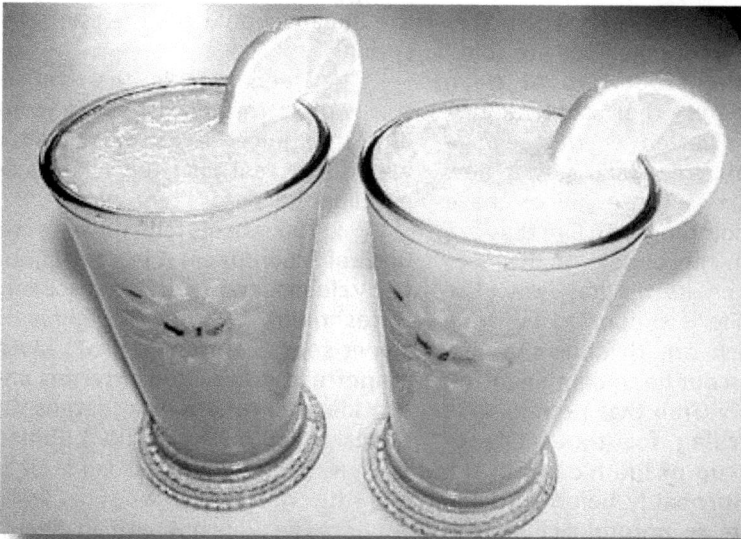

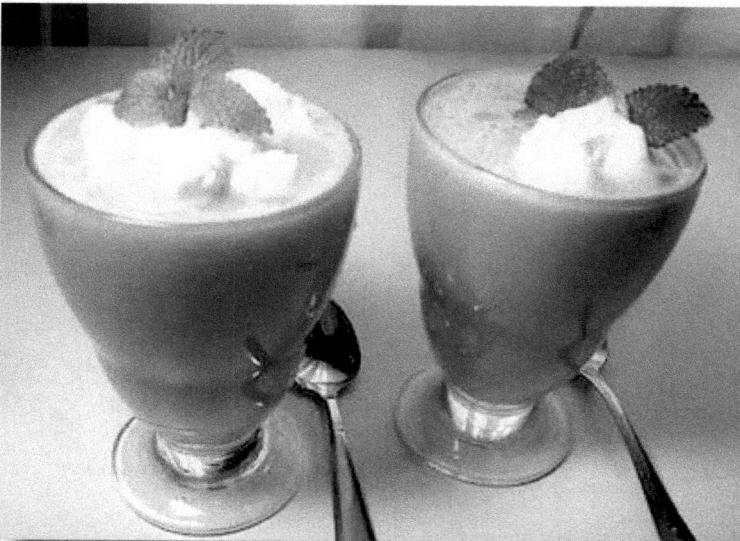

from freshly picked carrots has the highest quantity of life force. Even if we listed all the vitamins and minerals in a carrot, we could not describe the perfect balance they form together. If we listed all the diseases which carrot juice heals, the lists would be longer than several medical books. And if we wanted to explain why that is so, we could not because how could we explain life? **How would you explain the force that drives the world? Carrots are the engine of that force.** Vitamin A in the carrot complements vitamin C in tea, and that is way they both represent the recipe for the most important injection for the future.

Mango cocktail should be prepared with a juicer and citrus squeezer. We can treat ourselves by drinking sweet mango juice and nibbling on lime. Sweet wine is the real Jesus's wine, so serve it in chalice. One or two glasses of natural juice a day makes a great plan, but don't forget pure water...

In the near future there will be small wooden kitchen presses available on the market – a smaller variety to wine presses. These will be far handier than electrical juices, quiet, more efficient, the price several times lower than the electrical ones and clean in minutes. If you are interested when they will be available, keep informed on the news from the Medicine of Nature on the internet site.

Cocktails of the future: companies packing fresh, unpasteurized juices, with the shelf life of 2 days and highly frequent distribution. I have witnessed this practice on vacation in Poland and was pleasantly surprised. Not a day went by without me enjoying fresh pineapple, carrot, grapefruit or orange juice from the supermarket. At first, fresh juices will make their way to retail stores, then bars, inns and night clubs, where they will begin to make cocktails out of fresh juices. The array of fresh juice will increase, with only a little bit of alcohol in modern cocktails for the flavour and aroma. This is called healthy entertainment. Dj come and play my song...

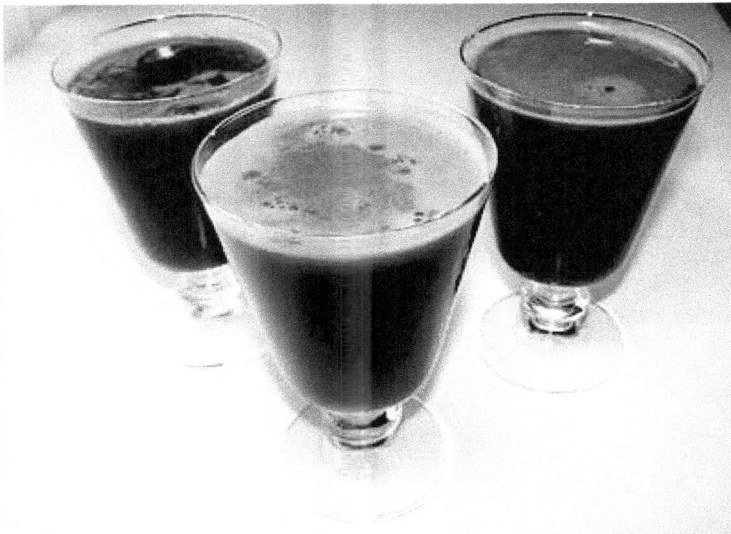

Vanilla ice-cream:
1 kg of peeled bananas,
2 dl fresh cream,
100 g dates,
1 dl pure water,
1 tbs of honey,
1 small spoon of
powdered bourbon vanilla

Chocolate ice-cream:
1 kg of peeled bananas,
50 g powdered cocoa,
2 dl fresh cream,
2 tbs coconut oil
or 4 tbs of coconut butter,
100 g dates,
1 tbs of honey,
1 dl pure water

Strawberry ice-cream:
1 kg of peeled bananas,
½ kg strawberries,
2 dl fresh cream,
100 g dates,
1 tbs of honey

Blueberry ice-cream:
1 kg of peeled bananas,
½ kg blueberries,
2 dl fresh cream,
100 g dates,
2 tbs of honey,
1 dl of pure water

Peach and apricot ice-cream:
1 kg of peeled bananas,
½ kg of peaches or apricots,
2 dl fresh cream,
100 g dates,
1 tbs of honey,
1 dl of pure water

Almond-hazelnut ice-cream:
1 kg of peeled bananas,
50 -100 g of almonds,
50 g of hazelnuts,
2 dl fresh cream,
100 g dates,
1 tbs of honey,
½ small spoon of vanilla,
1 dl of pure water

Coffee ice-cream:
1 kg of peeled bananas,
50 g of coffee,
1 dl of fresh cream,
30 g of coconut oil,
50 g dates,
1 tbs of honey

PREMIUM NATURAL ICE-CREAMS

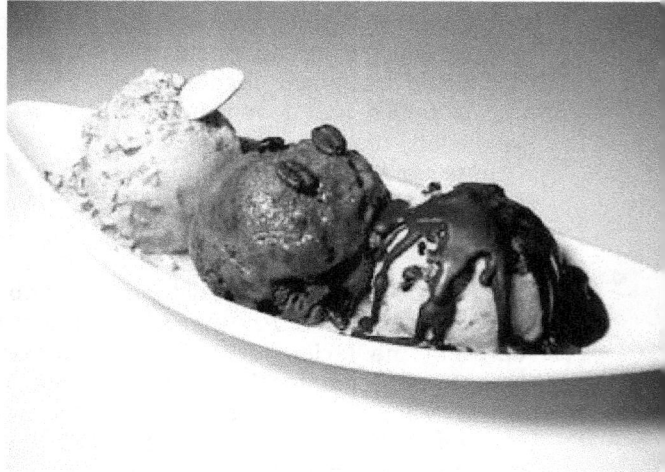

Technically speaking, ice-cream is a homogenous mixture of ice crystals, sugars and fats. I have studied several books on ice-cream technologies and it's all a big jumble! Homogenized milk, motor oil, artificial flavours, stabilizers, white sugar ... Why do we think this world is so advanced, when children can make better ice cream than the one made from all those formulas, graphs, tables and learned technical terms.

I was making and selling natural ice-creams one summer. I was using ecologically grown fruit, dates, cocoa beans, real vanilla...and I had a

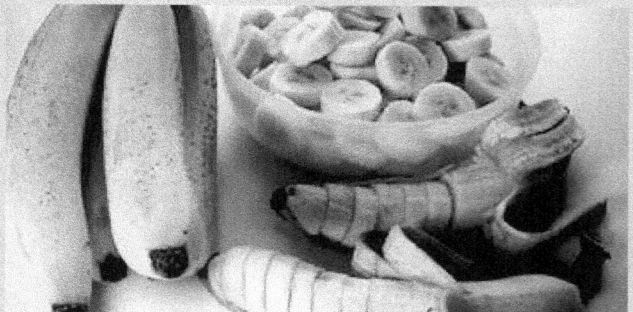

lot of enthusiastic clients. I have always been a dreamer. One of my wishes is to open a chain of natural confectionery shops all over the world's greatest cities. It might come true, who knows. It's about time, because industrial junk, which is advertised in such a big manner, is no refreshment at all, unless refreshment means heart attack and stroke? Real fruit, fresh cream, honey, and bourbon vanilla - that is real refreshment! I will give you some of the recipes from my brief ice-cream making career. In the beginning, you will find listed recipes and the technology follows. Preparation of delicious, healthy ice-cream is like a child's play. These recipies are based on bananas which are perfect for ice cream base because of sugar content and creamy structure, but there are also other types of healthy ice creams, one such is based on truly raw cashews...

Peel the bananas, cut them in pieces and freeze over night. Soak the date nuts in 1 dl of water for a quarter of an hour, whip the cream, cut the fruit and everything to the make ice-cream is ready. Mix the frozen bananas, soaked date nuts together with water, fresh fruit (it can be partially frozen), whipped cream, honey, vanilla in a blender and you will get creamy ice-cream. If you want to make scoops, put it in a freezer for several hours. The other option is to freeze all the fruit, which will make the ice-cream more compact, but also more difficult to mix. When preparing the almond-hazelnut flavour, grind all the nuts in a coffee grinder. Ice-cream decoration in an eternal classic: chopped up hazelnuts, almond slices, natural chocolate and cocoa beans. Child's play! Your refreshment is melting...

Bananas are a great foundation for natural ice-creams and if you don't like them, you can use truly raw cashew nuts. Vegans can use coconut oil instead of cream. Before "the best natural ice-cream in town" comes to your city, you can make it yourself and let your children help you. And by the way, premium is the designation for ice-creams with high cream content.

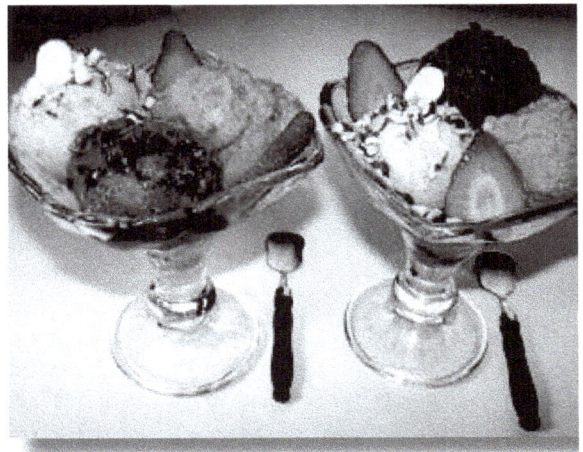

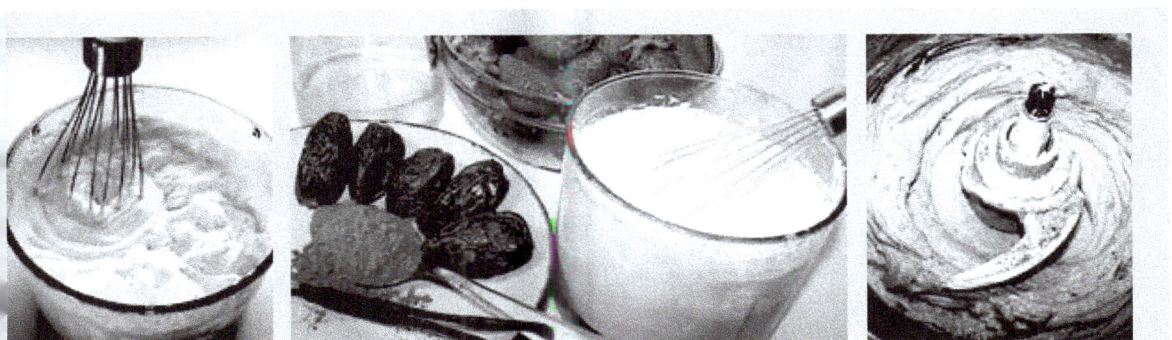

Figs in cinnamon chocolate:
12 dry figs,
6 tbs of grated
fresh cocoanut butter,
1-2 tbs of powdered cocoa,
2 tbs of agave nectar,
cinnamon

Plums with walnut marzipan:
12 prunes,
walnut marzipan:
6 tbs ground walnuts,
1 tbs coconut oil,
1 tbs honey,
chocolate icing:
4 tbs coconut butter,
2 tbs powdered cocoa,
1 tbs agave nectar

Dates stuffed
with cocoa beans:
12 dates,
12 whole cocoa beans,
4 tbs grated cocoa butter,
2 tbs powdered cocoa,
1 tbs of agave nectar

NATURAL PRALINES

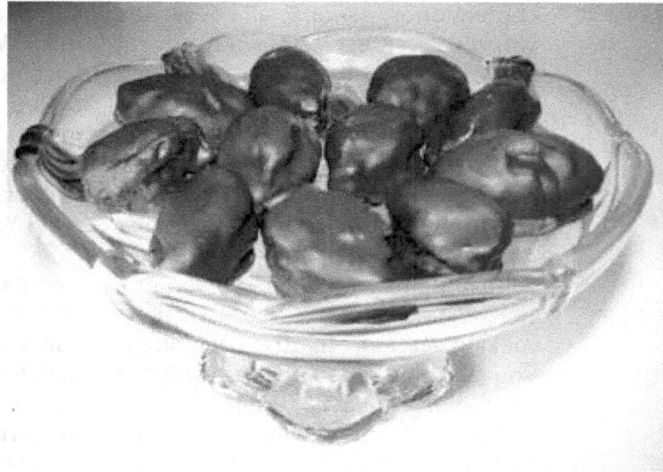

The nature is offering us luxury in abundance, but we twist it around and break it into pieces like hooligans, who decided to destroy a new car. We extract white sugar from the natural tree molasses, roast nuts, extract flavours, filter oils, break down, tear apart, separate, drain and then put back together. It's the story of Frankenstein. He's alive, he's alive, he's alive! I don't think so. Numerous artificial pralines are little Frankensteins.

Are you craving for sugar? We are saving the best for last; dried fruit coated with chocolate. Nature made everything perfect, why don't we use it as it is? Ok, let's make it a little better. Our lives will

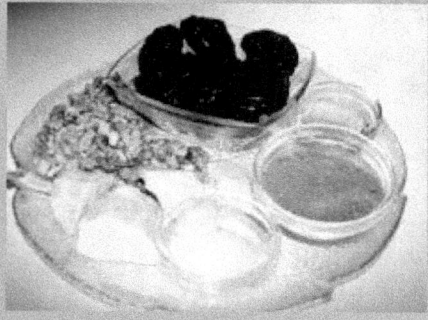
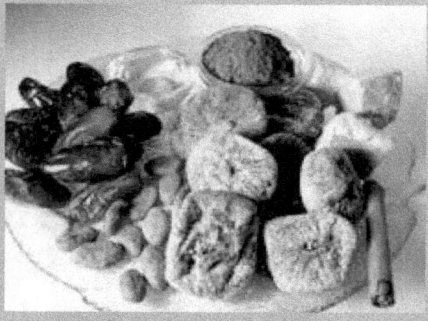
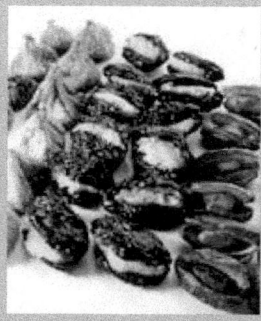
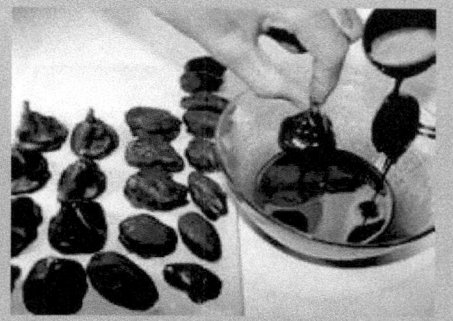

be sweeter, but not shorter. Research findings show that those who regularly consume chocolate in small quantities, live longer. **Chocolate is useful, but we can't say that it is healthy like we can say without any reservations for the fruit.** If we eat chocolate in moderation in small quantities it will benefit us, it might even prolong our lives because of the abundance of antioxidants it contains. Dried fruit coated with fresh chocolate are natural pralines par excellence, natural sugars covered with antioxidants. Perfection in a black tuxedo.

When we take a bite of premium prune, we hear gentle rustle of crispy seeds in natural gel. What more can we add? Nothing, thank God! Thank you Mother Nature! Shape the figs into small pyramids and put them in the freezer for about an hour; then prepare raw chocolate so the fig ladies can dip their behinds in the chocolate. Like a luxury seven-star spa resort.

Prunes yearning for pampering in luxurious hotel lie on the sofa. They spit out the pit and call room service. "Walnut marzipan, please!" Grind the walnuts and mix them with honey and coconut oil and serve the prunes with a teaspoon. They fill up their tummies until they are full and burp, and at that moment grab them and dip them into chocolate. Let them cool and when in the mood, enjoy the sweet bite.

The distinguished gentlemen, the date nuts have bladder stones. Gently cut them and replace them with whole aromatic cocoa beans. Keep them in the freezer for one hour so that the chocolate sticks properly. A bath of fresh chocolate prepared in a double dish is imminent, as well as relaxing on chairs covered with baking paper for at least two hours after surgery.

Here are few more ideas before we say goodbye. You should try and dry any fruit of the season, be that strawberries, apricots, peaches, figs, persimmon, oranges or mulberries, because it is almost impossible to find properly dried fruit on the market. Dried fruit in natural chocolate are real desserts, a pure fantasy. Look for your future here and you will find it.

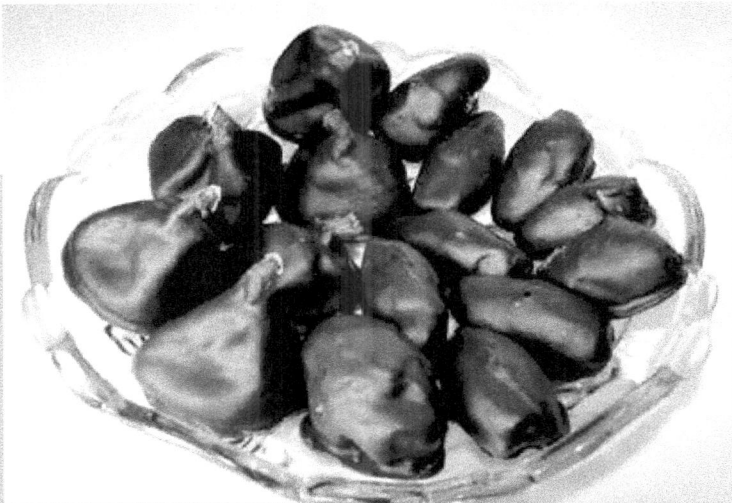

FOR THE END

Because life ends somewhere around 42°C, we will slowly conclude this book with 42nd recipy, although the recipes continue. There is no end here, these are only the new process foundations for healthy, intelligent cooking, so experiment as long as you are alive. Modify the preparation procedures and discover new tastes. Try to upgrade the recipies and improve the serving method. Live out your fantasies and **follow the principle – do not destroy life, glorify it!** Follow that principle and try to prepare some traditional or your family's favourite dish. If you discover some amazing new combination please share it with me so we can share with others as well. Keep in touch and regularly visit our web site www.Medicineofnature. com, where you will find more and more information on this healthy lifestyle.

NIKOLA TESLA IS LAUGHING

I would like to recommend you the book THE METHOD OF HALF-FASTING - The Alternating Current in Medicine, Medicine of Nature 3th book for further reading, which is expected to be released in future. **In the past, fasting has been perceived as a superior medicine with impressive effects, but we are on the threshold of new discoveries.** Semi-fasting is a universal healing method, which is easier and better than fasting. Semi-fasting means that we fast during the day by drinking water and juices and enjoy a moderate meal of fresh food in the late afternoon. The cycle should be repeated in 24 hours, as this provides the best rhythm for cleansing and recovery for the body. **Let's synchronize with the cosmos, with the 24-hour-long rhythm of the planet Earth.**

When transmitting electric energy, direct current can travel for only short distances, while alternating current can travel almost without any limitations. It is the same with semi-fasting; it can last a lot longer than fasting and it provides better results in the long run. Most people refuse fasting, because they equate it with starvation, but they have no problem with half-fasting. It is a fact that we do not starve when half-fasting, but rather that we eat like kings and queens. Taste sharpens a lot during the day and each bite of food we consume in the late afternoon tastes like never before, it tastes heavenly. Semi-fasting will be the central healing method in all the hospitals in the future. The secret is in the correct rhythm, which has magical effects on the body; it revives it. Detailed explanation will be provided in the book so eagerly expected by many, but you can get short instructions online also.

HEALING CHOCOLATLE

A book titled **Green Medicine and the New Herbarium – The Correct Use of herbs, Leaves and Green-leaved Vegetables, Medicine of Nature Part 4** is also in the works. It is based on studies done by numerous researchers like Ann Wigmore, Victoria Bouthenko, Victoras Kulvinskas, my personal and others, who draw attention to the deficit of greens in the modern human diet. **When observing the** monkeys, they have found that they are very strong and resilient, because they chew green leaves, which are not as appetizing to us, fine human beings, as they once were. The pharmaceutical industry produces extracts from different parts of plants, but by the time those get extracted, the active substances are already dead. Natural extraction of active substances from the green parts of plants is very simple, we only need a blender and a strainer.

One more recipe at the end. Chocolatle is a great ancestor of chocolate in liquid form. It is an old recipe from Mayan civilization. It was made from crushed cocoa beans mixed with water, cinnamon, vanilla, cloves, nutmeg and chilli. We will bring it back to life in the highly nutritional Chocolatle. We will make a natural extraction from the leaves of fruit trees: pear, apple, plum, hazelnut... or from a bunch of lemon balm. **Take a bunch of fruit tree leaves and blend it in a blender with a glass of water and then strain. Since their main ingredients, chlorophyll and magnesium are bitter, heaped spoon of cocoa shall be perfect for covering the taste.** Add a spoon of agave nectar and it is like you are on Yucatan. **The Mayan ruler Montezuma drank Chocolatle from golden chalices, which he allegedly threw away after drinking, because the drink had been so sacred.** If he knew the recipe for the therapeutic Chocolatle, he might have reached the old age of Methuselah and could have told us in person when the next solar eclipse is coming and why the World is coming to its **end**.

Special Appendix:

Reforms

All of the texts below you can listen spoken in my own voice on official internet site of Medicine of Nature: www.Medicineofnature.com, where you will be able to hear, see, taste and verify even more truth.

Sincerely yours,
Mathias Mark Sanderson

Medicine of Nature
Part One

Global Health Reform

Hello, my name is Mathias Mark Sanderson.I am an independent researcher, visionary, founder of Medicine of Nature and author of two books. After many years of research there have been discovered the most probable solutions, which can fix financial, healthcare and ecological crisis the world is facing, because all three are tightly connected. Actually my work is based on work of many other independant scientists working in the same field, but there are some new solutions – a very important ones.

In past five years I wrote two books named Medicine of Nature 1 and Medicine of Nature 2. The first book describes all you need to know for your personal health reform and also what the society has to do in order to heal. The book offers a plan for the global healthcare reform- the real one. It explains why orthodox and alternative medicines work only in a limited scope, or in other words; don't really work at all. Both books present the only way of natural healing with its most important and central factor - a properly composed diet or live nutrition.

Medicine of Nature is not a human invention it is an ancient, method of healing, actually most conservative one, which uses the power of natural forces only. The method is extremely efficient if applied correctly healing up to 90 % of modern diseases. When these methods will be accepted as a base of medical practice, our civilization will heal.

Natural healing began with Hippocrates and reawakened some 200 years ago under the name Natural Hygiene. Because hygiene means outer cleanliness, a new name was formed – the Medicine of Nature. This is a continuation of Natural Hygiene and a new generation of proper healing treatment suitable for wide use; not only for certain lucky individuals but for whole society. Due to numerous innovations and improvements, it has reached a mature form for general use and presents the stepping stone of the future healthcare and pharmaceutical system.

In short, let me present the first book of the medicine of nature. The book describes how humans have completely turned away from a natural way of life, which is the cause of modern disease. It describes what our food was like in ancient times and how we lived, when there were no diseases, which we know and suffer today. The book describes today's most common diseases and what occurs in the body stricken by them. Therein are explanations why the medicines don't work and what real pharmacy should be like - the green pharmacy; whose beginning of widespread use is only a matter of time. The book describes in detail the appropriate work of doctors in the future. Their work will be prescribing natural diet instead of pharmaceutical preparations. The task of a doctor will be the prescription of various forms of fasting instead of surgical procedures. Reading the book we realize that diseases which widespread medicine claims to be incurable; are in fact in most cases curable.

The book explains in details which food is natural and which is not. There are many foods categorized as natural food, but a great deal of what we nowadays define as healthy food is actually only healthy to a certain degree. A good example is whole-wheat or integral bread which is supposed to have a good, healthy effect only if consumed with a lot of fresh vegetables for example and in moderate quantities ofcourse. A vegetarian meal is only healthy if it is full of fresh living substances, in other words if it contains at least half fresh ingredients, by fresh I mean raw. Social misconceptions are a big obstacle on the road to health. The era of awareness has arrived and opinions will greatly change on what healthy food is and what healthy life style is or what it should be. Even more important than this is the change of the general perception of what is the correct way of healing, all of which is based on right understanding.

The book gives instructions to those seriously devoted to discover the truth; it is an exceptional source for politicians, medical staff, doctors, merchants, inn-keepers, caterers, managers, directors, media, chefs etc. The final chapters of the book are short but of a large format in contents – a true wealth of information. The book is carefully crafted giving links and interlinks in all spheres of human life, even architecture, because the high, shiny buildings are not an ideal place to live in. People are intended to live in nature as they were living in the past. If we could build skyscrapers we can restore our natural habitat as well. As inteligent beings we can build large parks and orchards to find peace, listen to the birds singing feast our eyes on the greens, and smell the blossoming flowers. In the parks around the towns we could build small eco houses each with their medium sized terrace

and large garden to grow fruit and vegetables. Sounds idyllic? No, this is the way it should be; this is the right environment for life. Listen or read a detailed description of green belts around cities in the audio recording no. 6.

Despite its fairly rich contents, the book is easy to read and even humorous at times to make it more pleasurable. A couple of hours of reading will change your life forever. By purchasing the book you will attain knowledge for life and at the same time give your support to the development of medicine in the right direction, since 90% of the assets from the sales will be contributed to the development of the project. Keep on listening to the next tape.

Medicine of Nature
Part Two

The Book of Recipies

MODERN HEALTHY GASTRONOMY

The second volume of Medicine of Nature – book of recipies is much more than just a cookbook – it combines medicine and gastronomy in a unique way. It is an innovative cookbook, first of its kind, which combines cooked and raw food, so that it cooks and bakes only food, which is inedible raw and leaves all the other ingredients natural and so preserves their vitality. It is a new way of cooking – smart cooking where most vitamins, enzymes and minerals remain preserved unchanged, thus supporting life. The book contains recipies for the most popular dishes in the world, but is aplicable universaly. This cooking procedures and techniques are different from what we are used to, the dishes made in this way are delicious, healthy, and the vitamins are truly preserved, not just allegedly preserved like we read they are in numerous new age cookbooks and newspaper columns. It is much more than a cookbook because it gives us the guidelines for the gastronomy of the future. It will influence profesional and amateur cooks, housewives, chefs, restaurant owners and most importantly, the food industry.

There is a common belief a healthy diet means missing out on eating dishes such as pasta with tomato sauce, chocolate pudding, pancakes with strawberry jam, or vanilla ice cream – a false assumption. This is now past time belief. We do not have to restrain ourselves from eating those popular dishes, we do not have to renounce, we simply have to prepare them in a different way. You will be surprised when you try your favourite dishes prepared according to these recipes and enjoy them without any feeling of guilt.

A SHORT HISTORY OF CULINARY ART

A short history of gastronomy tells us that humans in ancient times ate the same food as animals; food in its natural state, as it was found. After the discovery of fire many inedible foods became edible and the rate of survival has increased; but what followed was a mistake. We began to cook also the food which didn't need cooking at all because it was perfectly edible in a raw state e.g. tomato, pepper, carrot, spinach, fruits, walnuts, etc. Today almost everything is cooked - all ingredients fly into one pot. The modern culinary art, regardless of the number of stars awarded to a restaurant which pomposely hang above the entrance of that restaurant, is not something we can be proud of because more than 90 % of the dishes' vital ingredients are destroyed by temperature, while our body cells yearn for them, cells scream for vitality. In the numerous books on healthy living we read about healthy food but the recipes offered in those books denature the vitamins actaly destroy them. From a culinary perspective fire is useful in the kitchen, but the health aspect requires us to use it only for food which is not edible raw such as potatoes, peas, legumes, or mushrooms etc... we divide food into two categories; the one which we cook and the other we use raw. The recipes of the Medicine of Nature combine the ancient way of life with modern civilized ways, which is a very important combination made.

Recently, raw food diet has become fashionable and indeed it is definitely the best diet for one's health, but only a handful of people can live this way. In fact such a radical change is not necessary since up to 75 % of fresh foods in a diet is sufficient to fully suply body with live nutrients. But how to manage that, when we simply love that not so healthy food, such as pasta with tomato sauce? Cooked tomato is mildly toxic, a raw tomato sauce is healthy - a complete difference. The same can be said for spinach sauce and other popular recipies. Perhaps we could prepare fresh tomato sauce? Yes and incredibly good one, or two, or there,or four, five diferent, many actually. Every tomato sauce on the supermarket shelves can be made fresh. Whole-wheat pasta with fresh tomato sauce is from a health standpoint a completely different dish than pasta made from white refined flour with sauce from cooked tomato or even canned tomatoes.

The next excellent representative recipy in the book is apple strudel and walnut and poppy-seed rolls; bake only the pastry (the crust), then we cut it ahalf and fill it with different delicious fresh, raw fillings. The flavour of the strudel and rolls is even better while, at the same time, the body cells get the vital food they need. The 'know-how' is in the recipe book. I strongly recomend

you to try it out for your self. Smart cooking opens the door to healthy living for a vast majority of people.

The first recipy is very uncommon tea which can be used as an exceptional universal cure. It is made of rosehip powder. Rosehip tea is usually cooked or even boiled which destroys C vitamin in it. In this recipe we grind the rosehip buds into fine powder and pour warm water over it so the tea is at body temperature. If preparation is at body temperature, vitamin C stays fully active - 100%. Of course, the same as with classic rosehip tea adding lemon and honey is indispensable, but never in a hot tea – see the recipy. The Natural C tea, as I named this incredible cure, instantly relieves headache and clears the mind. It is far better than Aspirin because it is completely natural and has no side effects at all. In the future this will be the first 'medicine' you will get when admitted to a hospital because it instantly strengthens the immune system and mobilizes the internal healing forces. Natural C tea is excellent when you are facing any daunting task or mental work as it improves concentration and focuses the mind.

There are more good examples of the innovative recipes in the book such as marmalades without sugar made without cooking which are far better than those which are cooked with lots of sugar in a classical way. A great innovation are the healing soups so called because they can practically help to cure any disease. There are recipes for pies where you bake the crusts separately and then top them with fresh fruit, natural marmelades and/ or fruit from natural compotes. Similarly, for pizzas you only bake the crust topped with vegetables such as zucchini, eggplants, mushrooms, asparagus, artichokes, etc. After about 10 minutes of baking we remove the pizza from the oven and only now we top it with fresh tomato sauce, poure on some cold pressed olive oil, fresh garlic, sprinkle it with fresh basil and oregano, add some unpasteurized olives and capers on top and serve the pizza with grated fresh cheese or fondue. In this way basically all the ingredients apart from the crust and a few vegetables are saved from destruction by heat – see the book of recipies.

In our cookbook there are puddings, where we cook the rice in water and only after we add and mix other ingredients raw; the best puddings ever. Another good example is peanut butter with 30 % roasted and 70 % raw peanuts. What do you think it tastes like?It is very good. This peanut butter has no serious competition and it would be great if governments around the world and even better if public taste it. Also there is a recipe for natural Schweppes which tastes better than the original. The recipy for schweppes was the inspiration for natural Coca-Cola, which will be a drink of the future but this Coke will be blameless – a new experience and joy for young and old.

There are many more amazing examples as there is virtually no dish which cannot be made in a healthier way, you just only have to know how. You can turn these recipes into thousands of others; the important thing is to learn new technical procedures which preserve life – let this book be an inspiration for your favourite dishes maybe not for all but for certain surely. Health food enthusiasts will love it, many cooks and chefs all over the world will begin to adhere to the principle of vitality in their recipies, and the industry will pick up on these recipes when implementing new standards. These recipes will change the standards of modern gastronomy and development of the modern culinary art. The change will happen slowly, but it will reach everyone who cares about their heath. Firstly, It will reach health resorts and healthcare institutions, schools, restaurants, even fast food restaurants. But as always the change starts at home...

Method of half-fasting – the central doctor's tool

116

Now I will explain you the most important discovery in medicine in this century half-fasting , but first lets go to the roots. Fasting is an ancient method of healing which can produce incredible results. It strengthens the internal healing force, activates detoxification from head to toe, purifies the body, invigorates the immune system and all bodily functions and encourages healing of the wounds from the inside out. Fasting is a universal operation without scalpel; nonetheless to this day, it is not prescribed officially despite its efficiency. Why? Neglecting financial factors the reason is that fasting has its disadvantages. The first disadvantage is that it is hard to follow because renouncing food requires discipline. The second disadvantage is in the modern pace of life which is too quick for fasting. Food abstinence along with a lack of time exhausts the organism; so it is hard to follow while working, studying or carrying out other daily duties, because in ordinary fasting lack of energy is present all the time. The last, but not least disadvantage is the fact that noisy cities are no good places for fasting; in rest man needs peace, man needs a nice, quiet, comfy place to rest. Therefore the type of fasting we are familiar with is nowadays unfortunately only suitable for a handful of people in a specific environment under specific condition, not as a main tool in the future medicine.

THE MODERN FORM OF FAST FOR MEDICINAL PURPOSES

It is hard to believe that a better method of healing other than fast will ever be found, but we are on the verge of discovery. The fast has been recently substantially improved and the result is a new modern form of fasting, a fasting easier to follow, but with the same benefits – the half-fast. The half-fast is a siple and straightforward method but immensely beneficial as curative or preventive. It can be done by anyone, anywhere and anytime. It consists of drinking of pure water, tea and freshly squeezed fruit and vegetable juices during the day and one moderate meal of natural food a day prepared from natural ingredients. This one meal a day is slowly eaten in the second part of afternoon, any choosen time you like and prefer but meal should be eaten every day at the same time – this is important. The cycle repeats in 24 hours and gives the body the best rhythm for cleansing and rejuvenation. In this way we are fasting actually all day long, then break the fast and continue it the following day, break again and continue the next day. Excellent setting! This creates alternating current in the body.

The biological rhythms of our body are greatly influenced by the shift between the day and night and half-fast strengthens this biological rhythm. With 24-hour frequency also the amplitude of life increases; Breathing becomes deeper, heart beats deeper, life impulse is stronger, thoughts are clearer, etc.. Thanks to this rhythm, half-fast is even more efficient than fast. The 24-hour rhythm has exceptional power since within this period, all body functions normalize and the healing of virtually any disease is a normal consequence and is almost automatic, you just need to use a simple guidelines and switch to right frequency.

THE NIKOLA TESLA INSPIRATION FOR THE APPLICATION OF ALTERNATING CURRENT IN MEDICINE

Nikola Tesla was a great inspiration for aplication of alternating current in medicine. Some 100 years ago Nikola Tesla presented the alternating current to the world marking the beginning of the world's electrical power supply on a large scale - world electrification began Thanks to this invention, today, there is electricity in every house since alternating current can be transmitted to great distances, far away from power plant. This was not possible before with direct current, because power of direct current would fall drastically even on a distance of one kilometre, so efficiency to distribute electricity was low. For similar reason also in medicine we use alternating current. Nikola Tesla was a great inspiration because this type of current also has numerous benefits for use as a cure. We fast for 24 hours, then we eat a meal and fast again next day. Both phases alternate rhythmically and through the body runs alternating current with very low frequency - 24-hour frequency The main advantage of half-fast is

that it is straightforward, widely applicable and anyone can carry it out because of it's, we could say; 'natural simplicity'. People usually renounce and decline fast because for most it means starving but they experience no such problems with half-fasting method. Roughly estimated classic fasting is suitable for less than 5 % of people, whereas half-fast is suitable for 99 % of people.

THE ROYAL FEAST

The biggest difference is that during half-fast we are not starving, but in fact eating like kings and queens. It is a divine meal.The taste senses enhance during the day and each bite of food in the late afternoon is extremely delicious, food tastes like never before. If, while fasting, we are waiting and longing for the time to eat again, during half-fast we treat ourselves to a royal feast every day in the late afternoon.The food acquires a much better taste than usual, because the taste buds become very sensitive, the appetite is stronger, the healing is efficient and the patient enjoys the treatment.

A MATTER OF TIME

Because of these aforementioned advantages, half-fast is technically the most advanced form of fasting. Fast in this form is suitable for the modern age and it is only a matter of time when medical schools will teach the young generation of doctors how to properly conduct it and prescribe it to patients on a daily basis. Fast will be used in critical cases to quickly enable body for internal healing process to begin, whereas half-fast will be more used for chronic diseases. Patients suffering from critical conditions will be for example prescribed with a week of fast following with a month or two of half-fast. The cascade fast – half-fast will be employed to get the best of both methods. Half-fast can become the main method of healing in the hospitals of the future, it can change the medical science giving it the ability to become more effective and efficient than ever before. The secret of the recipe is the right rhythm which magically influences the organism and revives it.

THE GREAT MEDICAL EXPERIMENT

The day when a massive prescription of half-fast takes place instead of pills and surgery, will be a very nice day, probably sunny day. Many things will change in medicine. Natural medicines will be prescribed on every day basis; such as the green medicine, which we will explain soon, and natural C tea, with the core of the healthcare practice being half-fast. To introduce these changes, a great medical experiment is planned in the near future, an experiment which everyone can participate. Volunteers from all continents will test the method and gather enough evidence material for constitutional changes to occur.

Before commencing the half-fast, the patients will visit their doctor and request a general medical check-up. Medical examination will be done also after the completed half-fast and the difference of health condition will be a testament itself and fact recorded in many medical charts. When there are enough files recorded, the medical science will acquire the needed amount of evidence to begin constitutional changes. If you want to participate you can find and download the INSTRUCTIONS FOR HALF-FAST for free on the internet site of 'Medicine of Nature', in this way you will test and prove the efficiency of the method first for yourself. The cooperation is voluntary and at one's own responsibility. As the author, I believe that the method is completely safe and the very opposite of today's medical practices which are extremely dangerous. I invite you to participate in this great medical experiment and set for a journey that will forever change your life.

Health Reform
in the 21st Century

The health reform of the 21st century triggers a series of changes which are inevitable if we truly want to become an advanced and healthy civilization. In line with this reform the food industry, pharmaceutics, agriculture and education system will reshape and many more. The world will become a totally different place. Without this reforms, the crisis we face today is impossible to solve.

NEW FOUNDATIONS OF MEDICINE

The foundations of mighty medical structure will shake severely in the years to come and it will reform drastically. There are 10 million cancer victims per year alone and this indicates that the system is not effective and reform is inevitable. Why is it so? Because the foundations of medical practice are based on mistaken assumptions. Small doses of the so-called 'medicines' which are handed out to patients like communion in the church cannot cure an organism which is poisoned with artificial food. The presumptions are wrong.

If you ask the leading molecular biologists in the heap of DNA research how much progress has been made in the understanding of the functioning of the human body, they will reply not far at all. I quote the world's renowned microbiologist and ecologist David Suzuki. If you don't understand the operation of a machine, you cannot fix it – these are the laws; ask your mechanic. The understanding of the living organisms has deepened with the use of electronic microscopes but we can never control the complexities which we can observe with the naked eye with chemical substances. Only a higher intelligence can organize the internal processes and connect the body cells into one uniform operation capable of sustaining life.

The basic principle of natural holistic treatment says that the process of healing is driven by an internal healing force, not chemical compounds. Therefore the right treatment is creating conditions which activate the internal healing force; this force is the only one in authority for the management of biochemistry.

THE NEW HEALTHCARE PRACTICE

The new healthcare practice will be completely different than it is today with its starting point in the diet, not the pill. The healthcare reform begins with general practice – when visiting the doctor. Each doctor will be a highly trained dietician which will be a requirement for acquiring a university degree. Analysis of the blood, urine, listening to the heartbeat and lungs with a stethoscope, counting of the white and red blood cells, endoscopy and X-ray will be of secondary importance, because those analytical methods only measure the consequence but we are interested in the cause. The microscope will be examining the patient's plate. The doctor will ask the patient about his or her eating habits including what type of food is consumed and about the quantity and frequency of consumption per day, etc. Instead of counting calories as we do today, the nutritive value – the life value of food will be counted.

The main doctor's tool wil not be a stethoscope, scalpel or injection, but a pen and a block of paper. The doctor will listen carefully to the patient and record everything The notes will be a starting point where the treatment will begin The doctor's prescription will be a meticulously composed natural diet with the precision of a Swiss watch The basic recipe is going to be more or less the same, regardless of the disease – prescription of natural diet, prescription of fast or half-fast, prescription of drinking green medicine, natural C tea, fresh organic juices, etc.

The doctor will ask the patient about physical activities, the amount of sleep including afternoon rest, naps, sunbathing and other vital hygienic habits. Exercise and sports is taken seriously in new medicine because oxygen is the basic element of life and we acquire it in sufficient quantity only through movement The lungs which are the oxygen pump give the body full amount of air through movement and no other way. There is no life without oxygen The doctor will advise the patient on sports activities that should work best for every individual and patient and doctor will together make a yearly exercise plan. The doctor will advise and the patient will be actively involved in the treatment When they meet again they will reflect on the progress and adjust the treatment in accordance with the progress achieved. This is the correct procedure and the basis for treatment and prevention of any disease.

THE TEMPERATURE LIFE LIMIT 47°C– A FUNDAMENTAL PRINCIPLE OF FUTURE MEDICINE

The fundamental principle of future medicine is The Temperature Life limit which is at 47°C or 116° F. Enzymes in food are alive up to this temperature, for most food even lower, as much as 42°C or 107°F. The doctor will explain to the patient what is the principle of life in enzymes. He will explain the importance of combining the body enzimes with enzymes which are only present in living food. The joint work and assimilation of enzymes from both sides creates the flow of life. Enzymes in plants still function below 47°C – this temperature is the difference between life and death. In the desert however, there are only a few plants that thrive and survive on higher temperatures, because life in generaly ends at this point. But this plants have developed specific adaptations to sustain life, to keep enzymes active against all odds. Heat-processed food may seem the same as natural at the first sight, but if the enzymes in it are not biologicaly active, than the circuit of life is broken. The temperature life limit will be the center of future medicine, which will be after long centuries of misconceptions finally set on correct fundamentals, so this will be the most important topic between the doctor and the patient.

NEW PHARMACY

The foundations of today's pharmaceutical science are completely misguided. It is impossible to produce a medicine which would fit into the biochemistry of human body. Overly complex processes occur in the body to create an artificial mixture, which could fit into biological processes without any side-effects. Extraction procedures in use today obtain isolated concentrates which are biologically dead because of improper procedures. Besides, every synthetically made substance upsets the natural chemical balance of the body so it can be characterized as poison. The body needs living complexes - natural extracts created over many millions of years of evolution. Those substances are found in perfect mix in fresh vegetable juices and only these can be called medicine for man.

The doctor will only prescribe new medicines which will be made according to the principles of life. The production of medicines will use the same or similar processes as in the food industry. It will take into account the temperature life limit, because medicine, as described by Hippocrates, is nothing more than a highly nutritious food. The temperature life limit must be taken into account in the production of all medication without the use of chemical extractions, solvents, distillation, etc..only natural extractions. Depending on the available technological knowledge including computer science, this is not a daunting task as long as the technologist is lead by the right principles – sane principles.

The pharmacist all over the world compete and endeavor to discover a miraculous drug, mysterious in its functioning, but the one thing a modern man needs most is chlorophyll; a compound found in green leaves. Chlorophyll is a basic compound of life like air and water. The proportion of greens in the diet of monkeys is about 40%, in the diet of man it should be at least 20%. It is a shame that green leaves and young buds are no longer tasty to the modern - civilized people, but this now is a fact. Green leaves and young sprouts have been replaced with pasta, bread, rice, potatoes and other carbohydrates so people are severely lacking chlorophyll and other essential elements from green leaves: magnesium, calcium, iron, selenium, copper etc. Natural mixtures are allways complex, very complex and everything is needed, not only extract of a single component, because in the body it functions together. The extraction of natural medicines from green leaves is a simple and brilliant solution that can change the pharmaceutical disaster to an extremely successful healing treatment in the future.

THE EXTRACTION OF GREEN MEDICINE

It is so simple and in life only the simple things really work. You can prepare the green leaves extract, the true medicine at home, which is a big advantage. In a blender mix a bunch of green leafy vegetables with a cup of water. You can use wild herbs such as nettles or even tree leaves, fruit tree leaves, anything that is green is worth to try. With a few short pulses, the green plant complex is released, which we then strain and get a cup of green coloured drink, the best medicine in the world – **the green medicine.** The preparation requires only a few minutes. More guidance about natural extraction is given in the first book of Medicine of Nature.

MEDICINES AS FAR AS YOU CAN SEE

There are enough green leaves as far as your eyes can see, so this medicine is accessible to everyone regardless of how wealthy or poor one is, which is a huge triumph. It does not need special cultivation; it is available anywhere and anytime. Simply, take a look through the window at the forests and orchards – all of this is cure; the best in the world, and this really is the pharmacy that makes a difference – a pharmacy that works. Chewing medicinal plants is the ancient way of extraction and animals still use t today. Yet people have the intellect and kitchen utensils.

In the hospitals of the future there will be storages of fresh greens and the medicines will be made to order fresh, depending on the needs of patients. Different mixtures of plants will be combined to give a wide variety of medicines for specific purposes. The doctor will prescribe the daily doses and the intervals of treatments and the pharmacist will mix and extract fresh greens to produce the medicine.

MODERN SURGERY

The surgery will continue to progress but this invasive method will be used less and less. Instead of referring the patients to a surgeon; the general practitioners will, in most cases, prescribe fasting which activates the internal healing force. The treatment will begin with a short fast followed by a longer half-fast. This will be modern surgery without a scalpel. Along with the fasting daily doses of differen green medicines will be prescribed. As a result of fasting, the blood is diluted and therefore the medicine has a higher concentration in it, and so a greater effect. This is the correct way to increase the effect of the medication and not isolating individual substances and than concentrating them into pills which is a mistaken pharmaceutical procedure today. Modern surgery goes hand in hand with New pharmacy.

NEW LEGISLATION

The world needs a new legislation in the field of health care. A number of people are aware of the problems but they do not find solutions in a vicious circle and feel powerless in seemingly insolvable situations. The results of my research and many scientists around the world show that the solutions are on the horizon, they only need to be implemented in practice. All those who are listening to presented program of reforms are invited to actively participate - anyone can contribute something to find out the answers to the many; still troubling questions.

The health reform is the most important political topic for both; internal and foreign policy because the problem is global. It will bring about the greatest progress of civilization and improvement of quality of life globaly. If the health reform is carried out relatively quickly and efficiently, it will be a testament that the age in which we live is truly the age of science and knowledge and, particularly the age of common sense. The reform is close by; I invite you to listen to the next recording.

Changes in the
Food Industry

Even if the medical science reforms and doctors begin to treat diseases properly, we will still face a big issue because today's food is ruined by the way it is cultivated and processed; in the food we have on the market today there is basically very little life value. Doctors cannot prescribe healthy food if the industry keeps on producing refined oils, white sugar, white flour, pasteurized dairy products and cans by the million. If we follow the cause behind any illness, the trail goes back to the food factories. Why very little is done about this fact? Actaually almost an absolute lethargy! The government institutions have no real agenda; in fact, they have no plan for the future of all of us. The doctors' association should demand institutional changes for new standards for food processing; food technologists should be assigned with the task of finding new procedures and not using the information technology to play computer games. Some solutions you will hear in next few minutes but some are still to be found.

People say that they cannot afford healthy food; but the food which is usually served on the table, was healthy at one point; before it underwent destructive processing. When balancing the costs of artificial food which is today cheaper and natural food that is today more expensive, it has to be taken into account that each refinement requires investment into technology and the use of vast amounts of energy, so we live in a time of utter nonsense and we are aware of what is happening but still no action is taken. Our food should be 100% natural at the same price as cheap junk food. The life and

vitality in food is delicate, sensitive just like our skin – we can quickly get burned. Processing of food should be much more careful and a lot wiser. For this sake we should reintroduce the good old ways from the pre-industrial period. A change in technologies is quite simple; first of all we need an initiative to change the legislation, which would regulate food processing in food industry.

PHARMACEUTICAL PLANTS FIRST

On the one hand wrong food industry, on the other hand wrong pharmaceutical industry. When refining sugar, the microelements are removed, in the production of pharmaceutics, the same microelements are concentrated into pills. Food is not machine, which can be dismantled and reassembled, it is a far cry. Iron, magnesium, calcium, vitamin C in the shape of effervescent pills? Both of the above mentioned production processes are wrong because life principles are neglected.

The changes in technological processes have to occur primarily in pharmaceutical factories followed by the entire food industry chain. What will happen? If we regulate the food processing by taking the life principles into account, the need for the pharmaceutical production will decrease. However, we should keep it going in order to save jobs but we should start with production of vital medicines such as syrups, tonics, natural herbal bonbons and of course fresh medicine – green medicine, best of all. The belief in pharmaceuticals is strong, patients often demand pharmaceuticals and this is the reason why the production of pharmaceuticals should be changed to harmless, highly nutritious, natural, vital substances. People are used to 'magical cures', but are entitled to get them without side effects. In this way the pharmaceutical companies will continue to have business opportunities and the people will get what they pay for - health.

REFINED OILS VERSUS COLD PRESSED OILS

There are 400,000 miles of blood vessels and capillaries in the human body – the distance between the Earth and the Moon. Now, just imagine how thin these capillaries must be and how quickly they clog. Refined oil molecules have changed polarity, they are inert fatty substances and the body cells cannot use them as such, this is why they clot the blood vessels and cause cardiac and cerebral strokes and so on and so on…. So, why do we keep producing them? These 'motor oils, as I named them, can be used for 20 and more times in a deep fryer. Do these oils even deserve the name food?

The press is a millennium-old device and it is all we need in the oil industry. Today's presses work with greater pressure than in past times and the efficiency is more than enough. The transformation of oil industry; refined oils into solely cold pressed oils is the easiest change of all technological processes

in the chain of changes and can happen practically overnight once we democratically decide to do so. Prohibition, historically speaking, has not been the most successful decision, but is definitely the right one for refined oils in other words we should only and solely produce cold refined oils for the sake of public health.

WHITE FLOUR VERSUS WHOLE-WHEAT FLOUR

Refinement of white flour is about 200 years old. Degradation of grain by removing its shell and sprout is in line with the development of modern diseases. On one hand you can find white flour on the shops' shelves and on the other hand, there are separately packed bran meals in the health food stores. Does it work? Of course not! White flour is just as deadly as white drugs, but the governments of the world are doing nothing about it. The minimum action to be taken by the governments to bring about changes is straightforward. Most people with whom I have discussed about various ideas of how to approach this issue, agree with the following proposition. The currently fairly high tax for foods made of 100% whole-wheat integral flour should be lowered by half. The food with lowered tax rate should be labelled as 100 % whole-wheat flour with no additives. As a result of this simple effort, the use of white flour would decrease. Then follows a series of other actions of which most important is price equalization; the same price for white and whole-

128

wheat flour products so that 'healthy stuff' is affordable for all, after being valued as a trendy and expensive for a short period in history. Since the regulation of lowered tax rate for whole-wheat products would still be in force, a wholesaler would make more money from selling whole-wheat products and would offer it more than products made of white flour. The third stage of actions is legalisation of higher prices for white flour than for whole-wheat flour. Consequently, white bread would once again become a commodity only for the richer as it was in the old times.

Prior to all these actions, there is but the most important new law, that should be adopted. As far as the food and health is concerned, this law could cause a turning point in this millennium. This law would state that every product on the market today made of white flour should also be available from 100 % whole-wheat, integral flour so that a consumer can make a decision and buy healthy food anytime, anywhere. Also in restaurants this regulation should be in force, so the customer would have a choice, everywhere. This law would be further replicated into every branch of the food industry; progressing with the dairy products which would be available in two varieties: pasteurized and unpasteurized. Once again, the consumer would be given the choice between healthy and unhealthy. Later in the development of the health food industry, pasteurization and refinement would be abolished, but these are steps that need to be taken before that. A reduction in the consumption of white flour would

have far-reaching consequences; substantially improving people's health in the long-term perspective. Gradually, we would change the general paradigm and people would begin to perceive white flour as a risky food, belonging to the same group as tobacco and alcohol. Then, one fine day in the distant future, white flour would only be a forgotten mistake of humankind.

WHITE SUGAR VERSUS RAW SUGAR

The most significant difference between white and brown sugar is the colour. Neither have microelements, vitamins or life which food must contain to serve it's purpose – sustain life. By the way, manytimes we find label raw on packages of sugar, but it is misguiding, this sugar is far away from raw. The first passive action here is the introduction of new labels on the basis of the temperature boundary of life, which will have a consequence that from all packages of brown sugar natural and bio labels will fall of until new, life-friendly processing methods without refining and heat will be discovered and employed. Then we can again attach different organic, natural, bio labels to brown sugar, this time justified. The annual global production of 1.7 billion of tons of refined sugar is a huge problem. We need to find a way to process sugar into crystal sugar considering the temperature boundary of life. One very simple and immediately implementable solution is to gradualy convert most drinks into healthy drinks using freshly squeezed cane juice as the base for the drinks – a naturally sweetened water. In the countries of the northern hemisphere fresh sugar cane juice could be done on the spot on the streets in bars, pubs like it is the case in some countries in the southern hemisphere. The bars, restaurants and other places that serve drinks could offer drinks made with fresh cane juice. Most important conversion of all; manufacturers of soft drinks should produce all the different drinks they produce now but on a base of fresh sugar cane juice instead of refined sugar and water. Of course, this would mean a completely different frequency of distribution because of short shelf life of drinks – but this is the only way to tackle the health problems on a large scale; there is no other way –this is the only possible and workable solution and we have to change or we will have the same rate of diseases in the years ahead as we have now- absurdly high rate.

The actions have to start in the parliaments; with the appropriate decrees which would jeopardize the free enterprise; which has turned into savage capitalism and is affecting society in a bad way. We have to adopt common sense policy, the trade legislation has to match natural legislation. Trade laws will have to be reassessed and reconciled with the laws of nature. We will have to organize transportation of freshly cut sugar cane to the Northern countries instead of crystal sugar. From a medical perspective it is a correct action and from political perspective likewise it is the only correct action Freshly pressed sugar cane juice can

have many more uses for example the ice cream industry as we will discuss shortly.

Despite these ideas, there is a great market demand for crystal sugar which we have become accustomed to and which is also far more practical for use. The sugar industry is in a desperate search to find new ways for processing crystal sugar at low temperatures. This is an open invitation for all scientists and innovators to come up with new ideas. Yet another issue with regard to sugar to think about; the North should pay a much farer price to South for the sugar cane and only in this way we could achieve a good economic and political balance of the world. At the same time, it is predicted that due to higher prices of sugar, the consumption of homemade dry fruit would increase in the confectionery industry. Thus, it is a win-win situation as dry fruit contains the ideal mixture of sugars, vitamins and minerals.

PASTEURIZED DAIRY PRODUCTS VERSUS NATURAL DAIRY PRODUCTS

Pasteurization is one of the greatest mistakes in history, because it is deadly for both microbes and humans. The little kittens die after being fed with pasteurized milk after only three weeks and the same would happen if we fed a baby with pasteurized mother's milk. The pasteurization process in the food industry is a mistake and should be corrected. As emphasised earlier, the temperature boundary of life at

47⁰ C and lower, should be respected in every process of milk industry; cheese, butter, cream cheese, etc. Thermal processing required for certain types of cheese can only go up to this temperature. The microbes are a part of the ecosystem and we don't need to destroy them providing that hygienic standards are maintained on a high levels, the cattle is treated in a humane way, and the market is supplied with fresh dairy products on daily basics.

The distribution system for natural dairy products is simple; cooled milk in bottles is delivered to the shops every day fresh. If it is not sold within 48 hours, it is returned to the factory, where cheese or cream cheese is made from actually still fresh and unchanged milk. Cheese made of raw milk is excellent. If it is not sold, it is ripened into mature cheese. This cheese has a shelf life of 2-3 years or more and the market price for it is higher every year. If by chance the deluxe mature cheese is not sold, it can be shipped by the Red Cross to Africa or other areas hit by some sort of crisis instead of powdered milk as is the case nowadays.

Raw butter can last for 2 weeks in the refrigerator and 2 months in a freezer. The same shelf life applies to cream meaning that these products can be used for quite a long time. Yoghurt and kefir follow the same sequence of procedures- cheese made from kefir is delicious. One major part of the new milk industry program is the mandatory increase of goat milk consumption, which is more suitable for human metabolism than cow's milk and has a much more suitable chemical composition for a human organism.

MARMALADES AND COMPOTES

Marmalades and dry fruit compotes as I describe them in the book of recipes are 100 % raw and thus healthy and because of their simplicity and excellent taste have the potential of becoming the new standard of fruit processing. Any marmalade or compote on the market today could be made by this method. The fruit is dried at low temperatures for 24-48 hours, packed and distributed and the consumers can make their own marmalades, jams or compotes. For all those, who can't find the time there are local companies which make fresh marmalades lasting for about a week. The marmalades are frequently delivered to stores, schools, kindergartens, hotels, government institutions, bakeries, confectioneries, etc. In bakeries fresh marmalades are added to the pastries after different types, kinds and shapes of pastries are already baked. For example, whole-wheat croissants are baked and only then filled with fresh- natural- nutritious marmalade. They can also be filled with raw chocolate, hazelnut or vanilla filling as I will explain in the next paragraph.

SPREADS, CREAMS, PUDDINGS AND CONFECTIONERY INDUSTRY

Today's hazelnut and chocolate spreads made of refined fat, white sugar and roasted hazelnuts are delicious but toxic. When I see children eating bread with Nutella or similar spreads I feel frustrated and guilty because we adults should take responsibility but very few people care about. People care about money, but they don't care much about responsibility.

There is a simple solution. With the use of a stone mill which has been used in ancient times for olive oil pressing, sweet spreads could be made without roasting. Stone mill is as useful today as it was in ancient times. Very slow grinding makes a silky smooth paste from any nuts and cocoa beans in 24-48 hours and, with the addition of natural sweeteners the paste changes into undisputedly healthy and wholesome spreads. Natural spreads and marmalades served with integral bread are the future and breakfast revolution. Nutty butters will be an inspiration for fairy-tale cream fillings in the confectionery industry. Imagine cookies with healthy creams, pancakes, cakes, puddings etc. in a healthy form, enabled by the old processing technique – the stone mills. The entire confectionery industry will change completely if we get the old mills turning yet again. Mills will turn and turn and slowly turn the whole confectionary industry.

CHOCOLATE AND CEREAL BARS

Let's shortly describe the new technological processes in the chocolate alchemy. We need to understand that most ingredients in the manufacturing of chocolate could be thermically unprocessed.

Cocoa butter should be cold pressed out of cocoa beans, and only than the cocoa beans could have undergone roasting process before grinding to cocoa powder in order to obtain the Maillard reaction, which gives the chocolate its specific caramel taste. Hazelnuts, almonds and peanuts do not have to be roasted; only dried at low temperatures in order to achieve crunchiness. Each chocolate bar needs to have the percentage of fresh ingredients labelled; ranging from at least 75 up to 100 %. In order to match the taste of healthy chocolates with the chocolates on the market today, the food technologists will have a lot of work but it is the only way to convert chocolate industry into healthy one .

As far as mueslis, energy and cereal bars, they could be made from cereal of sprouted grain, unroasted nuts, fruit dried at low temperatures, honey and healthy raw chocolate. Why destroy cereal bars with steam, roasting the nuts, glucose syrups and stabilizers? I think that this presented outlook of this part of the industry is extremely stable.

ICE CREAM INDUSTRY

The sweet juices sourced from sugar cane, palm flowers, coconut, birch and maple trees could be frozen fresh, transported by ships and used in the ice cream industry as such. Maybe ice creams could be produced directly on the ships. Of course cooling of large quantity of liquid is not cheap, but it is definitely cheaper than treating the health-destructive consequences caused by invert syrup and white sugar. Why to thicken tree juices by boiling them first, only to transport them and than again mix them with water into a sweet product latter in the factory? Nonsense! With the process of freezing the entire spectrum of ingredients is preserved as well as the vital value of the juices. Also the natural tree aromas are preserved so there is no need to add artificial flavouring because naturally flavoured ice creams are delicious.

The best ice creams are made of fresh fruit. But to make ice cream out of season, we can freeze a certain kind of fruit as we can freeze unpasteurized sweet cream. By separately freezing the ingredients we avoid preservatives. We mix the ice creams and pack them just before shipping them to the market. Why using the artificial vanilla flavouring, when powdered vanilla is 1000 times better? Healthy chocolate, unroasted nuts and cones made of whole-wheat flour and the children and adults alike will hardly wait for summer.

TOMATO SAUCES AND KETCHUPS

The preparation procedure for natural tomato sauces and ketchups is simple and described in the book of recipes. All different tomato sauces can be made 100 % healthy only the frequency of delivery to the stores has to be high because the packaging cannot have a due date of 1 year or more, but only maybe a week or so. It would be best to deliver the sauces fresh every 48 hours, however this is not necessary. It is incredible how almost

everything can be achieved; all that is needed is a new business practice and new legislation. It all starts with right understanding.

THE MEAT INDUSTRY AND FAST FOOD

In the post-war period meat was served only once a week and nowadays it is consumed frequently, every day. The increase of meat consumption is positively correlated with the increase in cancer and heart related diseases. Medical studies show that a vegetarian diet is far better in all aspects than a meat diet. Nonetheless, the promotion mechanisms for vegetarian diet which should be led by the governments all over the world are still very inefficient or non-existent. The production in meat industry has to be reduced by at least 100 times which implies an intensive advertising of vegetarian food. If people eat lots of meat, they don't eat enough fresh fruit and vegetables. Besides vegetarian diet is much more diverse, tasty and full of aromas –it is a kings diet.

Fast food can get much better than today. Integral bread, organic vegetables and natural ketchups and sauces would be a turning point for a new fast food standard. In sandwiches a little thinner slices of bread and a bit more fresh vegetables can make a difference. Every little thing can contribute and improve health standard. With a stone mill, mentioned earlier in the topic on confectionery, one can make vegetable spreads from sunflower seeds and different nuts. There are hundreds of very good recipies but none of those is used on a large scale in chain fast food restaurants. There are many good recipies for spreads even healthy mayonnaise and tatar sauce can be obtained with cold pressed sunflower oil and sunflower seed paste. A very good spreads are made of raw artichokes, cold pressed olive oil and different herbs. There are so many recipies, but when we enter fast food restaurant none of those is found, only standard refined junk food. Why?

PICKLED VEGETABLES

When pickling vegetables all that is necessary is the sterilization of jars, the equipment used and water whereas the vegetables should be raw; nor cooked nor pasteurized. Salt, pepper, vinegar, garlic and different spices are the best preservatives since ancient times. See recipies in the book.

REFRESHMENT DRINKS

In Poland there is a company which delivers fresh juices on daily bases made from apples, oranges, grapefruits, carrots, celery, pineapple, rhubarb, etc. The life expectancy for these juices is two days and the success rate of the company is huge. Also some other countries have this sort of offer, but the problem is that it is relatively small compared to the 'classic' junk, which takes more than 99 % of the market. Another possibility is healthy cocktails made from fresh juices in the bars, even perhaps with a small percentage of added alcohol to get the real cocktails but relatively healthy one. This new age cocktails should be promoted by barmans all over the world and young could encounter them on every party- sound party. Good practices are the messengers of the new age. Every country has some type of a good system in force which can spread globally – this is in fact the right process of globalization.

A very good practice is also the abolishment of plastic bags in Italy. From as little material as 20 plastic bags there is no problem to make the lifelong packaging of different dimensions that can circle between producer and consumer all the time. Reintroduction of recyclable glass bottles instead of plastic ones is another step which will change the attitude towards limited resources and the environment and build the future code of conduct. We have to raise awareness of limited resources on earth and change our behaviour. The best option would be to introduce recyclable packaging for all products – a big issue for the politicians to consider.

THE DIAMETRAL CONTRAST

Temperature boundary of life in the production of medicines and food will be registered in history as a great scientific achievement, like pasteurization was in the previous century, only that it is the complete opposite. There is a great deal of procedural solutions yet to be found and the course is already set – in the presented program of solutions.

In the next audio recording,

'Planet of Nature – Green Belts around the Cities' there is a plan for the setup of a modern human ecosystem. Although it sounds paradoxical that green belts around cities wouldn't create a huge profit, but they are actually the only solution to the global financial crisis and there is no other.

Planet of Nature— Green Belts around the Cities

From an evolutionary point of view it has not been long since we were truly the population of nature. We lived among the vast plant and animal kingdom and the tree tops and tree shadows and caves were our natural environment. The modern life takes place in a noisy, stressful cities where the tempo of life is way too fast. People are aware that life in the city is not the right way and a lot of people are moving back to the country, but this is a solution only for a minority of people who are not bound to work, studies or other city activities. There are some minor alternative solutions like ecological farms and eco villages, but the society still requires an integral solution for each and everyone. This recording offers a suggestion of a grand format. The quickest way to return to a natural way of life is to form vast parks on the outskirts of cities. Parks ranging to several kilometres wide, encircling the cities could solve many problems of the modern society. But, I don't mean parks as we know them today which are merely decorative walking grounds, but actual habitats for food cultivation, a place to live in and breathe with nature, very close to the city centre, within a stone's throw.

ORGANIC FOOD FOR EVERYONE

The heart of the project would be the cultivation of organic food under the slogan 'organic food for all'. The park would supply 100% organic food to all the city's inhabitants which would be the beginning of highly developed society, healthy society.

If we think about it from another perspective, not only would the parks offer healthy food, but a new culture would stem from it.We would re-establish a good relationship with the earth which feeds us and restore the systemswhich we depend upon and not the least we would develop much better social relationship and conduct, crime would decrease to unbelievable degree. Today's educationsystem is not founded correctly and the young generation is barely contributing to the society. We need education system in which student through work learns the basics of life and studies at the same time 'higher sciences'. Numerous orchards, crop beds and vegetable tunnels would offer the young a chance to learn basic survival skills. In close contact with nature they would learn a great deal about it and the co-dependency of people with all living creatures. At the same time they could provide for their families. If we can learn from little kittens, we see that they learn how to catch mice within several months, whereas people need 10-20 years to become independent and in many cases subsequently unemployed. Although professional specialization has increased, the primary basic survival skills have been forgotten. An active contribution to society has to start early and the precious knowledge of self-sufficiency means true independence for life.

THE SOLUTION OF THE ECONOMIC CRISIS

The economic growth has

reached its climax nonetheless; we are on our way down. Analitics say us China and Indian economy are good today, but is it waering masks in Calcuta or any big Indian or Chinese city a sign of prosperity? Dirty a r more dangerous than smoking tobacco and bottled water is a misunderstood economic sign. From the right point of view the econom c growth does not reflect progress. Monitoring of economic indicators and correcting the existing legislation cannot solve the world's econom c crisis. The solution lies somewhere where the majority of economists, analysts and politicians don't expect to find it. It lies in some really good recipies. The world needs a new social and cultural order. The large, passive majority of the population has to begin to contribute to wider society; in the first place the young population and at least 10% of the unemployed in the second place. In the developed world only 2-3% of the population is producing food which is far too low thus contributing to use of so many toxins while growing food. We have to grow If we want a healthy society at least 10% of the population has to grow food because organic food requires so many hands. Organic agriculture can save the human population, cure it from diseases, re-establish the balance of the ecosystems in nature and this is worth more than all the wealthof all the banks in the world combined.

Self-sufficiency is better than provision of social benefits; we just have to organize it at national and/or local levels. The ant societies have traits of both capitalism and socialism. Each ant carries something on its back, they communicate well among each other and each has its particularassignment. All those on benefits would keep them until the park starts to make profit so that they have money and food. There might be respectable housing in a natural surrounding for some diligent workers in the park, god bless them, as an alternative to renting places in cities at a high cost. Primarily, the food would be grown for our own needs and the rest would be sold in the park, fresh organic food would be sold at the same location as it is grown and city inhabitants would know where to buy a good stuff. Also, the city dwellers would visit the restaurants surrounded by the idyllic natural setting of the park, restaurants where only healthy food would be served. Because young students of life would prepare the meals and in this way learn the art of cooking which keeps all life value in the food untouched this meals would be sold at a low price affordable to anyone. With skills and knowledge the taste of healthy meals would be superior and even important citizens, government, managers and leaders would often come to have a 'business lunch' or just to rest in the beautiful surrounding. Additional income would come from tourist apartments in cottages in the best locations of the park, places so beautiful that would attract both local and foreign tourists. Also the touristic code of behaviour on such paradise locations would change, conscious rising everywhere in society. This is a brief description of the solution for the economic crisis. People need work which enables them to enjoy the basic commodities of life and to reconnect with nature, to live the full life again.

BIO-DIVERSITY, HEALTH CENTRES, BIO HOUSES, ELECTRIC VEHICLES, AMPHITHEATRE AND HEALTHY ENTERTAINMENT

We would plant different varieties of fruit trees, fruit bushes and other vegetation in the parks. Bio-diversity would be incredible. We would grow vegetables, outdoors in the summer and in greenhouses in the winter. The goal is biodiversity and botanic variety. Exceptional efforts would be made for growing the old apple varieties. We could grow all of the 5000 known varieties of apple trees, 500 known pear varieties, numerous different coloured apricots, peaches, kiwis, hundreds of kinds of tomato, strawberry, berries,etc. Certain parts of the parks would remain wild or almost wild for the animals to coexist in parks with people. If we manage to create a peaceful and non-violent culture the animals would stay in the parks and create a rich diversity which would fill our hearts with happiness.

In the park, there would be countless paths and creeks with wooden bridges; surrounded by small bio houses made of natural materials such as wood, stone, clay and straw. The houses would be relatively small because people do not need much indoor space anyway, but the verandas would be quite big and the gardens even bigger. This is an architectural plan which reduces the use of natural resources and save them for future generations. The houses would be designed to efficiently capture the solar energy

and to provide comfortable living spaces showered with sun light. We would use all the knowledge available for living in balance with nature and the whole park would run on solar energy. Every house would have a water tank and a basement for food storage which is far better than any refrigerator because it preserves the aura of life around food which stays touch with earth unaffected and so food has a longer lifespan and retains original taste. The houses would be leased on a time share basis to those who work in the park voluntarily with some people residing permanently. All those working in the park would be entitled to benefits in accordance with their contributions. People would have choices either to live temporarily or permanently in the park. This kind of life and freedom would appeal to many people, for some it would be a place of permanent residence whereas the others could come and go to park whenever they would like. People principally need food, shelter and clothes, but the park would offer much, much more.

The park would be a centre for health and recreation. It would offer a variety of playgrounds, sporting grounds and a lake for swimming in the summer and skating in the winter. However, the most popular recreation for all visitors including tourists would be gardening.The equipment made of materials such as wood and stone for exercising would be accessible to all and it will be used outdoors on fresh air which is a big advantage. Some would find it funny and say 'just like 'The Flintstones', but idea is really great because many can not afford the entrance fees for fitness gyms. Great idea, as it would be affordable to whole family rather than only individuals.

There would be no car admitted to the park; they would be parked in parking spaces before the entries to the park or on the exit roads from the city. There would be no lawn mowers, motorbikes sprinklers or any kind of noise but silence interrupted by pleasant birdsongs. We would meet only pedestrians and bikers on walking paths with some reserved paved roads for small vehicles powered on electricity.In brief, we would build a human natural habitat in a modern form.

There would be an amphitheatre built in the park for cultural events such as music, theatre performances, speakers and show of all kinds. It would be built out of stone and wood, like in the good old days; no plastic.

We would revive the old crafts such as pottery, glassblowing and knitting, the manufacturing of clothes using old techniques production of natural cosmetics and a number of local crafts. The park would have one big economical goal —self-sufficiency.

Small confectionary houses bakeries and cheese factories would be a model for the food industry as they would make products in accordance to the principles of life Children would learn how to make healthy chocolates, desserts,ice creams, natural cheese, yoghurt etc. It sounds like a fairy tale, which it is. It would be wonderful to take the kids for a Sunday getaway to the park and once they become adult, they could tell their children about their experiences when they were adolescents.

NEW GENERATION OF HEALTH CENTRES

A new generation of health centres will grow on the outskirts of the cities because oxygen is an immensely important element of healing and there is plenty of it in forests. The sick need peace, quiet surrounding and breathing in the embrace of the forest, where the natural homeopathy of scents accelerates the self-healing power. The eyes need the colours of nature; they need a rest from the computer screens and the green colour of nature has just the right frequency to usher serenity. Only the emergency rooms would remain in the cities whereas hospitals would move to the outskirts of the cities. Medical staff would learn about natural life, healthy food and fasting.The patients would help in the park according to their abilities during their recuperating stage because gardening is one of the best forms of recreation as involves natural movement. Where the air is pure, where there is peace and birds singing, where there are burbling creeks, where natural food grows and where people can live with nature, is where they should live.

MODEL FOR THE NEW ERA

The park would be a model for the new age which would reconnect people with nature. This is something completely different than the modern shopping malls. The greens instead of concrete; fresh air instead of exhaust fumes;quiet instead of noise; work instead of despair; health instead of illness;and the colours of life instead of the grey clouds. In fact we need the shopping malls just as much as we need parks – one completes the other. The green belt around the city would function as a large dynamo generating flow; the city as one pole; the park as the other pole and the flow between the two established. People would be only a step away from nature where they could catch their breath at the weekend, rest and then return to the city life. They could regularly charge their batteries. They could take a mini break every week with a minimum amount of time and causing minimum pollution. We don't have to travel thousands of miles when it is great to be at home. We also wouldn't have to transport the food over great distances, which would have a positive effect on people's health and the environment and a large part of the overall ecological problem would be solved.

The Dawn of the Healthy Civilization

When I wrote an article about the Planet of Nature for a paper some years ago, I got the reply that the idea of such a park is pure utopia. My answer was that if people lived in such a park and heard about life in cities, they would undoubtedly say that that was pure utopia. The second time around the article was published. There is some doubt whether the project could be feasible but if we were able to build gigantic skyscrapers and large glass shopping malls one after another;why shouldn't we be able tobuild parks of nature – one after another? No doubt.The biggest problem in the beginning would be to get the people enthusiastic about the idea because the park would be non-profit; but more useful to the society than all the shopping malls in the city centre together. Each great solution also has its difficulties, but if we face them head on, they become insignificant with time.

We are waiting for a city which would be the first to plant the green belts. The initiative has to come from the city council, the mayor or the inhabitants of the city. In order to build it, there needs to be a referendum. When the action would get underway, all the inhabitants of the city would get involved;primary schoolchildren, students, fire fighters, architects, gardeners, ecologists, mathematicians, construction workers, sellers, tourist workers, craftsmen,etc. The first such action will be one of the most positive projects in the recent history. The economic and healthcare crisis will soon only be a memory. The new values will be taught which will have the respect and the responsibility towards the planet at its core giving us a promise for the future.Tourism would develop in a tranquil form and we would leave behind proper cultural heritage for the generations to come.

The government authorities have to assignspecific rights to the cities required for the green belts to be built. The project will quickly prove successful and the enthusiasm of the inhabitants of the first city will excite the next larger city which will also take this great step. The first parks will deliver the objectives of the projectsuccessfullyand will soon spread around the world marking the beginning of a new civilisation. The basic plan for a park would be the same everywhere but the execution would differ according to climate, geological and cultural differences. The cities would become independent and self-sufficient and exchange of knowledge, people and various crop species would develop. The nature parks would be connected by long-distance trails in the unspoilt nature and numerous hikers would walk them every year marking the anniversary of the day when healthy civilization began. Perhaps a fairy tale, but this is the real Holly – wood.

Planet of Nature— Green Belts around the Cities

The Fields of Diamonds is a true story, which happened a long time ago and reflects the current state of the world.

THE STORY OF FIELDS OF DIAMONDS

Once upon a time, when the Earth was still flat, not far from the river Ind lived a farmer by the name of Ali Hafed. He was a rich man. He had a substantial part of land, where he grew fruit trees, vegetables, flowers and decorative bushes. He did well, as his gardens of eden gave him much more than he needed to provide for his family. He was a content man, because he was rich and he was rich, because he was content.

One day a Buddhist monk, one of the wise men from the East, came to visit him on his property. When they sat by the fire in the evening, the Buddhist monk began explaining how the world was created to the farmer Ali. "The world was once an endless, shining white and cloddish haze," he began telling his story. The Almighty in the beginning stretched out his hand and circled with his finger until the fog began spiralling. It span faster and faster, became thicker and achieved such velocity that it instantly turned into a fireball. The fireball circled around the universe and turned all the haze it encountered into steam, the downpours of rain, which fell onto the red-hot surface cooled it, formed the hills and the valleys, desserts and oases of our beautiful planet. The Earth was born. The fire rivers from the centre of the planet slowly hardened into granite, copper, partly into silver, a little into gold, and just a little into diamonds. The diamonds are the condensed drops of sunlight," mysteriously added the monk. Farmer Ali listened attentively. "You could buy up all the land around the river Ind if you had a diamond the size of a hazelnut and if you had a diamond mine, you could rule the country. Your children would be respected and esteemed all over the kingdom," continued the monk.

That night Ali went to sleep feeling miserable. For the first time in his life he slept like a poor man. Not because he lost anything, but because he was dissatisfied. He wanted the diamonds, a whole mine of diamonds! First thing the next morning, when he woke up, he asked the monk, where he could find the diamonds. The monk asked him, "Why do you need diamonds?" 'I want to be rich,' was his answer. "Well, then go and find them! That is what you have to do. Go and find them and you will have them.' The farmer lowered his eyes and said, " But I do not know where to look for them!" "If you find a river that runs over white sand in between two tall mountains, you will find the diamonds in the white sand, " said the monk. "I don't believe that such a river exists,' doubtfully remarked Ali. "Oh, there are many such rivers,' said the monk,' all you have to do is go and find them and then you will have the diamonds."

This is how Ali decided to sell his property, the orchards, flower plantations and the beautiful blossoming bushes. He began his journey to the unknown world in search of diamonds. He walked from Palestine all over Europe, from river to river, over hills and valleys, but could not find diamonds anywhere. He walked endlessly and used up all his life energy, but had no luck. He reached the Barcelona Bay at the end of the world known at that time, without any money feeling depressed and exhausted from searching the shiny pebbles. From all the grief and sadness he gazed into the upcoming wave of the ocean. He dived into the next wave. He disappeared forever in the foamy waves of the heavy waters, which were his last place of comfort...

Meanwhile at the other end of the world the new owner of Ali's gardens joyfully watered the plants and gathered the crops. He put his delicious fruits into a basket, decorated them with flowers and took them to the market to sell or trade them for other goods. One day, as he led his camel to one of the streams in his new gardens, he noticed a strange flickering of light on the sandy bottom of the shallow water. He took a small black stone from the water, which had a small eye reflecting in all the colours of the rainbow. For quite some time he curiously gazed at the stone and admired it. He put it in his pocket, later placed it on the window shelf and forgot about it.

Shortly after this event the Buddhist monk came to visit him and when he saw his find, he exclaimed "A diamond! A diamond!" "Where did you get this diamond?" he curiously inquired the new landowner, "Has he by chance returned?" "Oh, no, he hasn't returned. I found the stone in one of the streams in the gardens," replied the new landowner. Filled with excitement they both returned to the place, where the stone had lain and poked with their fingers into the white, sun bleached sand and to their surprise found another stone and another and another – there were so many...

This is a true story of the discovery of the diamond mine Golconda, one of the largest diamond mines in history. The English and Russian crown diamonds come from this mine.

The lesson of the story is far richer than all of the diamonds in the mine. **Abundance lies within us, the treasures that lie before our feet – pick them up.** All the wealth, richness, abundance is always within us; we simply need to be aware of it. **The powers of healing are within us and only those powers can cure us.** If we seek health elsewhere, we will lose our life, as Ali Hafed lost it, but if we place our trust into our plot of land and cultivate it with care and intelligence, we will become rich. We will become health millionaires, far richer than all the millionaires in the world.

I have adapted the story from the story-telling of Russell Crowell, who told the story in the previous century all across America in front of wide audiences, over five thousand times in a row.

To those who wish to live in a better world; who have any kind of suggestions, knowledge, skills, competences or ideas which would benefit the project and to all who believe that they can develop the suggested projects and who support the project by purchasing the books, woluntary work & donations, are invited to join. How? Spread the idea, talk about this important subject with others, or if you have a specific suggestion or idea, contact me personally.

Anyone who wishes to contribute to the development of the project should do so by purchasing the books. Those who wish to contribute a larger amount should order a larger number of books and distribute them among friends and by doing so, support the project in the best possible way and spread the information. By ordering more books you not only support the project financialy but at the same time spread most important part of reinaissance– knowledge of life for life. The project should be brought to a constitutional stage; but before that the information has to spread by translating the books into world languages. To sum up; read the books, use the recipes, support the project by purchasing the books and see you in the planet of nature.